Frontline Treatment of COPD

Snowdrift
Pulmonary
Conference

A Monograph for Primary Care Physicians

Frontline Treatment of COPD

Second Edition

The Authors

J. Roy Duke, Jr., M.D.	West Palm Beach, FL
James T. Good, Jr., M.D.	Denver, CO
Leonard D. Hudson, M.D.	Seattle, WA
Dean D. Mergenthaler, M.D.	Palm Beach Gardens, FL
John F. Murray, M.D.	San Francisco, CA
Thomas A. Neff, M.D.	Denver, CO
Thomas L. Petty, M.D.*	Denver, CO
Donald R. Rollins, M.D.	Lewisburg, WV

*Editor

First edition 1996
Second edition
2000

The Snowdrift
Pulmonary
Conference is a
function of the The
Snowdrift Pulmonary
Foundation, Inc.
A New Jersey
Nonprofit
Corporation

The Snowdrift
Pulmonary
Conference
1850 High Street
Denver, CO 80218

Printed and bound in
the United States of
America.

ISBN 0-9671809-3-7

Contents

Figures

Tables

We dedicate this monograph to the late
Thomas A. Neff (1937 to 1994), our beloved colleague.
Tom was a consummate physician, a great husband and
father, and a tremendous human being.
We shall always be enriched by his memory.

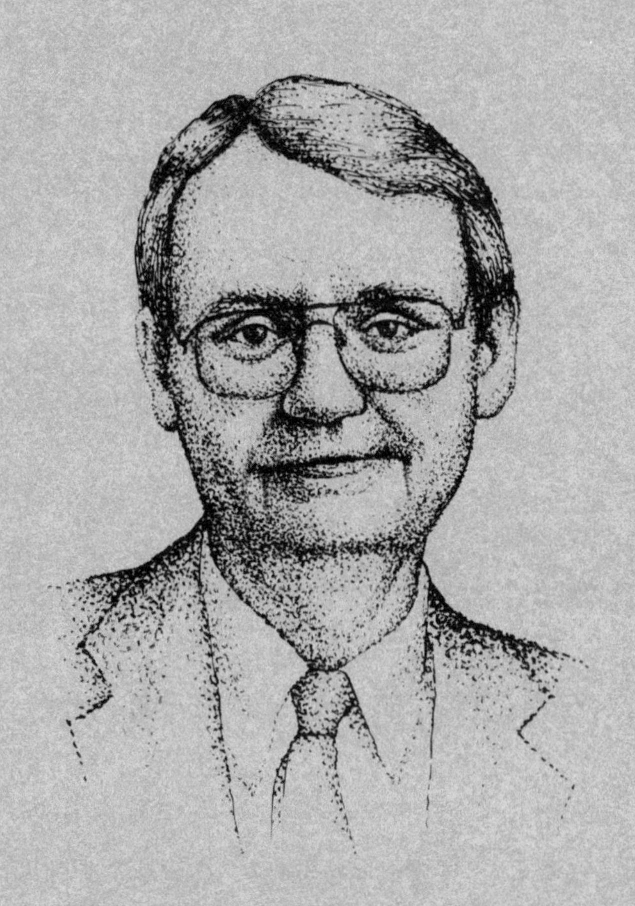

Preface

The first edition of *Frontline Treatment of COPD* has reached more than 100,000 frontline practitioners. This monograph has been used extensively in postgraduate education programs for internists, family practitioners, nurse practitioners, physicians' assistants, pharmacists, clinic and office nurses, and respiratory therapists. *Frontline Treatment of COPD* has been the subject of Grand Rounds in several university hospitals and many community hospitals around the Country. Many of the authors of the first edition have participated in these continuing medical education programs.

In conjunction with Medical Education Resources, fall programs held on Saturday mornings have been well attended, and the program, based upon this monograph has been extremely well received. The sponsors have also produced a two hour audio tape that carries the major messages of this monograph.

This monograph was first published in 1996. In view of significant advances in our understanding of the pathogenesis of COPD, new developments in pharmacological management and experimental surgical approaches, it became necessary to produce a second edition. A new national healthcare initiative, the National Lung Health Education Program, (NLHEP), aims to involve all primary care practitioners in the early identification and intervention in COPD. Section M of this second edition describes the NLHEP and its goals and objectives.

In the past, we learned to treat acute respiratory failure, to improve the quality and length of life with ambulatory oxygen therapy, and to increase the horizons of patients suffering advanced respiratory insufficiency through the development of pulmonary rehabilitation programs. Now it is time to take a hard look at preventing the progress of COPD when it is diagnosed in early and often asymptomatic stages.

The Editor

A. Summary

The term chronic obstructive pulmonary disease, (COPD), refers to a group of respiratory disorders, including chronic bronchitis, pulmonary emphysema, and asthmatic bronchitis, that nearly always coexist to varying degrees. COPD causes clinically significant progressive obstruction to expiratory airflow.

COPD is a common and important disorder. It is the fourth most common cause of death in the United States. In fact, 30 to 35 million Americans are believed to be afflicted, about half of whom are symptomatic.

The pathogenesis of COPD is becoming better understood. Currently accepted concepts include a progressive inflammatory response, possibly associated with unrestrained proteolytic enzyme release and toxic oxygen radicle production, induced by cigarette smoke and other inhaled pollutants. Why only 15% to 20% of cigarette smokers are predisposed to develop COPD remains an important unanswered question.

Many details about the natural history of COPD are lacking. But it is clear that susceptible smokers have an accelerated rate of deterioration of expiratory airflow compared with other persons, and that smoking cessation restores the rate of decline to normal.

Patients who are symptomatic or who have chest x-ray abnormalities resulting from COPD generally have moderately severe or advanced disease. In other words, the typical symptoms and signs of COPD occur late in its evolution. Patients with early COPD are often asymptomatic or nearly so, and diagnosis can be made only by documenting the presence of expiratory airflow obstruction. Simple spirometry is all that is required, and should be available in the office to screen all heavy smokers and other persons at risk for COPD.

The management of COPD is not difficult, but it requires a thorough evaluation of all aspects of the patient's illness and the thoughtful implementation of a treatment program that can be revised as needs change. The goals of therapy are to improve symptoms, to minimize deterioration of lung function, and to prevent hospitalization. These can be attained by a four-phase management strategy:

a. Smoking cessation and patient and family education about COPD.
b. Treatment of all reversible components of airflow obstruction using drugs selected from a hierarchy of available agents. Oxygen therapy and exercise are important adjuncts in advanced disease.
c. Early treatment of the precipitating causes of acute exacerbations in the outpatient setting.
d. Prevention of non-COPD complications of therapy.

Among the intercurrent complications of COPD, infections are the most frequent and important. These usually present as acute purulent bronchitis, manifested chiefly by increased cough, sputum production, and dyspnea often without fever, leukocytosis, and new chest x-ray abnormalities. Empirical antimicrobial therapy with amoxicillin or trimethoprim sulfamethoxazole is usually successful. Pneumonia is apt to be clinically more severe. A search should be made for the causative microorganism and specific therapy administered. Otherwise, broad-spectrum antimicrobial treatment is indicated.

Patients with COPD are at increased risk for postoperative respiratory complications. These can be minimized by preoperative preparation, careful perioperative management, and most importantly postoperative care, including particular attention to maneuvers aimed at restoring the patient's ability to cough and take deep breaths.

(continued)

Transient nocturnal oxygen desaturation is common in patients with COPD. Usually it is caused by sleep-induced respiratory physiologic abnormalities and not by classic sleep apnea; the mechanism can be identified by physiologic monitoring during sleep. Treatment with supplementary oxygen appears to be warranted, but definitive indications will depend on the results of future studies.

Acute respiratory failure represents a life-threatening deterioration in the course of COPD that is caused by an intercurrent complication, usually acute purulent bronchitis or another pulmonary infection, but possibly oversedation, surgery, or congestive heart failure. Confirmation of the diagnosis requires arterial blood gas analysis. Oxygen therapy is essential while all other aspects of treatment, including administration of corticosteroids, are intensified. Intubation and mechanical ventilation are needed in only a minority of patients (10%), but are lifesaving when indicated. The prognosis is better than customarily believed, and the patient's lung function generally returns to its previous baseline level.

Cor pulmonale, also known as right ventricular dilation or hypertrophy secondary to lung disease, is a late complication of COPD. It occurs earlier in patients whose airflow obstruction is caused predominantly by chronic obstructive bronchitis than in those who suffer chiefly from emphysema. Depending on its severity, right-sided heart failure in patients with COPD-associated cor pulmonale is treated with a progressive regimen of salt restriction and diuretics, followed by continuous oxygen administration.

Pulmonary rehabilitation is a method of integrated multidisciplinary care that offers improved well-being and quality of life to many patients with advanced COPD. The components of pulmonary rehabilitation, which are added to routine medical therapy, are:

a. Patient and family education.
b. Smoking cessation.
c. Systemic exercise.
d. Breathing training and respiratory muscle exercise.
e. Oxygen therapy in selected patients.
f. Patient support groups.

These strategies are now also being offered to patients with early COPD who may also benefit from them.

Most cases of COPD are caused by tobacco smoking. Smoking cessation is the only tactic guaranteed to slow the progressive decline of expiratory airflow that culminates in COPD. It also minimizes the risks of acquiring many other deadly smoking-related diseases that kill nearly half a million persons in the United States each year. Primary care physicians play an important role in ensuring that their patients stop smoking. Always ask if patients smoke. If they do, advise them to quit. Suggest that they take advantage of the many available community resources to quit smoking. Arrange follow-up for reinforcement. It is difficult to stop smoking, but with the proper advice and encouragement, it can be done. ■

B. Definitions

COPD is an all-inclusive and nonspecific term that refers to a defined set of breathing-related symptoms: chronic cough, expectoration, varying degrees of exertional dyspnea, and a significant and progressive reduction in expiratory airflow. Most patients with COPD are smokers.[1]

Airflow obstruction does not show major reversibility in response to pharmacologic agents. Hyperinflation and a reduced diffusing capacity may be present. Inflammatory damage to both airways (bronchitis), and alveoli (emphysema), is found upon postmortem examination.

COPD is an umbrella term used to encompass several more specific respiratory conditions that may exist individually or in any combination. The terms chronic obstructive airways disease (COAD), chronic obstructive lung disease (COLD), chronic airflow (or airways) obstruction (CAO), and chronic airflow limitation (CAL) all refer to the same disorder. The specific components of COPD are as follows:

Chronic Obstructive Bronchitis

Chronic obstructive bronchitis can be found in patients with cough, expectoration, and diminished airflow that does not improve significantly after bronchodilator inhalation. Simple chronic bronchitis, or chronic cough and expectoration with normal airflow, is not included in this definition. Simple chronic bronchitis without airflow obstruction has a good prognosis, and there is not such a severe social and economic impact on patients, their families, or society. (Chronic obstructive bronchitis is distinguished from asthmatic bronchitis, discussed below, only by its lack of reversibility in response to pharmacological agents.) Patients with

1 The definition of COPD has varied over the years. Today it includes ICD-9 codes for chronic bronchitis (491), emphasema (492), and other chronic airways obstruction (494-496). Isolated asthma, particularly reversible asthma (493), is not included.

pure chronic obstructive bronchitis do not have physiologic or roentgenographic evidence of hyperinflation. Diffusion tests are normal or nearly so.

Emphysema

Historically, emphysema was defined pathologically as reduced elastic recoil and the disintegration of alveolar walls due to tissue breakdown through the processes summarized in Section D. Clinically, emphysema patients exhibit varying degrees of dyspnea upon exertion and irreversible airflow obstruction. These patients also demonstrate abnormalities at the air/blood interface that manifest in decreased carbon monoxide uptake (measured by diffusion tests) and hyperinflation (judged clinically by physical examination, x-ray, and measurements of total lung capacity). Chronic bronchitis and emphysema, of course, usually coexist because both are caused by tobacco smoking. Most clinicians continue to use the term "COPD" for this reason.

Asthmatic Bronchitis

Patients with asthmatic bronchitis have pulmonary symptoms, including productive cough, exertional dyspnea, and airflow obstruction, but these symptoms and the obstruction reverse significantly in response to inhaled beta-agonists, anticholinergics, methylxanthines, and corticosteroids (used either alone or in combination). In these patients, progressive airflow obstruction occurs over time and becomes less reversible.

Diagnosing asthmatic bronchitis in its early stages, when airflow abnormalities are just beginning to occur, may be profoundly important. In both asthmatic and chronic bronchitis, bronchial hyperreactivity probably results from airways inflammation caused by a variety of irritants (including smoke). This hyperresponsiveness is likely to reverse significantly if the patient stops smoking, avoids other irritants, and uses bronchodilators. The regular use of bronchodilators or inhaled corticosteroids in the early stages of disease may help forestall or prevent irreversible damage and may make impairment, disability, and death from "endstage" COPD less likely.

In their later stages, chronic obstructive bronchitis and asthmatic bronchitis may become indistinguishable. Therefore, airflow obstruction that is chronic, progressive, and partially reversible in response to bronchoactive drugs is the key indication of the bronchial component of COPD. ■

References

Petty TL, Hodgkin JE. Definitions and epidemiology of COPD. Chapter 1 in Hodgkin JE, Petty TL (eds). *Chronic Obstructive Pulmonary Disease: Current Concepts*. Philadelphia: WB Saunders, 1987. This chapter presents useful clinical definitions for COPD.

C. Epidemiology

COPD is now the fourth most common cause of death in the United States. It is the only cause of death among the top 10 that continues to rise. In 2000, there will be approximately 115,000 deaths from COPD. In 1994, there were 500,000 hospitalizations, 14 million office visits, and 114 million patient days of restricted activity from COPD in the United States. The medical costs from COPD are also increasing among the elderly population.

COPD can be considered a smoker's disease that clusters in families and worsens with age. The hereditary patterns that contribute to COPD have not been identified, except in the case of alpha-1-antitrypsin deficiency (Discussed in Section D).

The risk factors for COPD are genetic, constitutional, behavioral, socioeconomic, and environmental. Tobacco smoke and occupational hazards, when present, should be eliminated since they are the two major external factors that can be altered. However, constitutional risk factors cannot be changed. It has been estimated that 80% to 85% of COPD cases in the United States are attributable to tobacco smoking. In addition, smoking cessation slows the decline in expiratory airflow. This clearly shows that smoking or its cessation is a powerful factor determining a patient's outcome. Other contributing factors in COPD include air pollution, childhood respiratory infections, and nonspecific bronchial hyperreactivity.

Morbidity and mortality from COPD are more common in whites compared with blacks, and in men compared with women. Figure 1 presents the death rates for COPD by age, sex, and race in the United States in 1997. While the number of men who die from COPD annually is beginning to drop slightly, the number of COPD deaths in white and black women have increased steadly since 1980, probably because of increased smoking in this group (See Figure 2). The

Figure 1 1997 COPD Deaths by Age, Sex, and Race

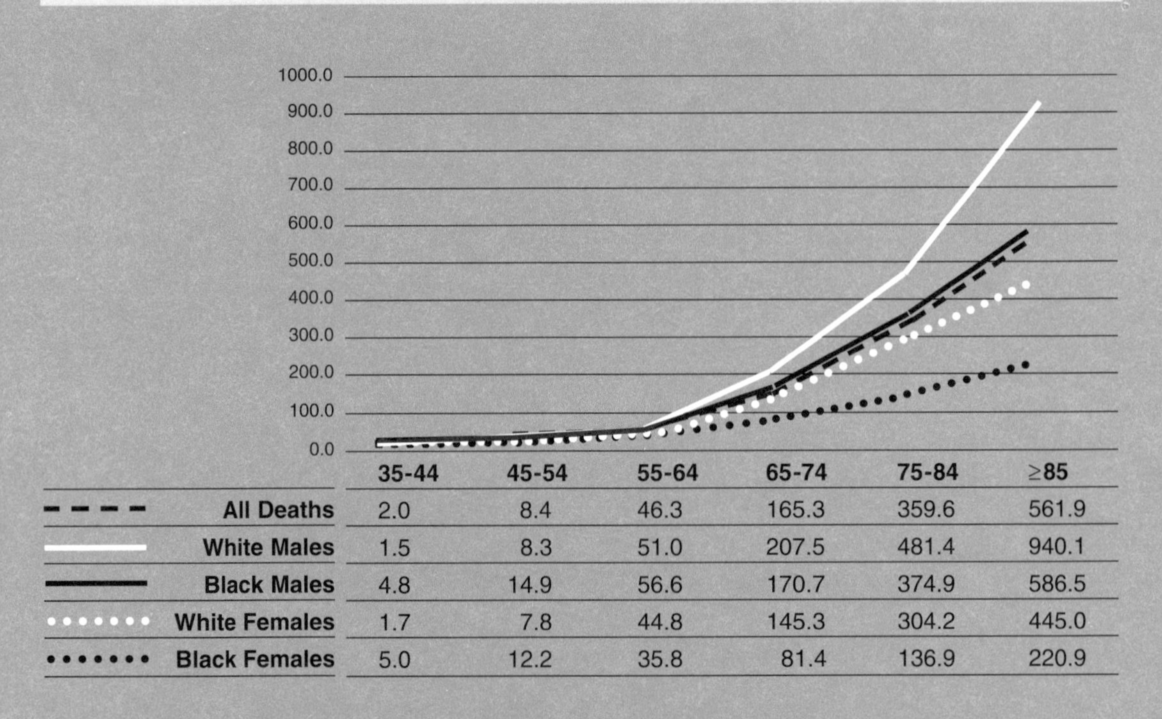

	35-44	45-54	55-64	65-74	75-84	≥85
All Deaths	2.0	8.4	46.3	165.3	359.6	561.9
White Males	1.5	8.3	51.0	207.5	481.4	940.1
Black Males	4.8	14.9	56.6	170.7	374.9	586.5
White Females	1.7	7.8	44.8	145.3	304.2	445.0
Black Females	5.0	12.2	35.8	81.4	136.9	220.9

Figure 2 COPD Deaths/100,000 by Year

	1980	1985	1990	1995	1997
All Deaths	15.9	18.8	19.7	20.8	21.1
White Males	26.7	28.7	27.4	26.6	26.5
Black Males	20.9	24.8	26.5	25.4	24.5
White Females	9.2	12.9	15.2	17.8	18.5
Black Females	6.3	8.8	10.7	12.5	12.7

Source for Figures 1 and 2: *Health,* United States, 1999. U.S. Department of Health and Human Services. Centers for Disease Control and Prevention, 1999 DHHS Publication #99–1232, p.179 to 180.

Figure 3 COPD Death Rates by Country, Sex, and Age (35 to 74 Years)

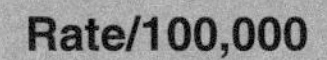

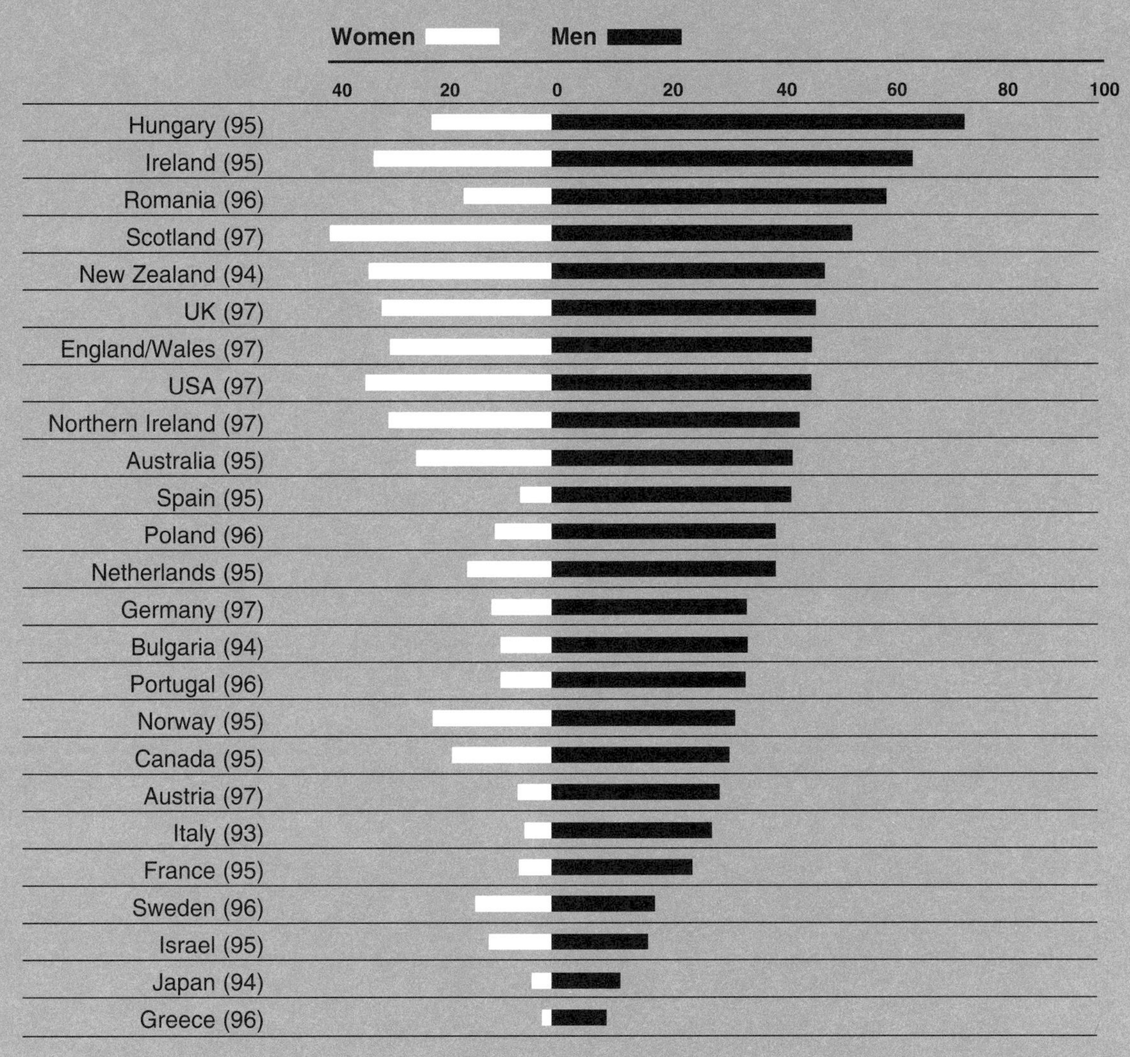

Age-adjusted death rates for COPD by country and by sex, ages 35 to 74 years (adapted from World Health Statistics Annual, WHO, unpublished).

prevalence of COPD in developed countries is similar to that in the United States. Elsewhere in the world it is not well defined, but limited data from Asia (particularly India and China) suggest a high prevalence of the disease in these places (See Figure 3).

At least 16 million persons in the United States have symptomatic COPD. The third National Health and Nutrition Examination Survey, (NHANES III), estimates that at least another 16 million people in the United States have asymptomatic, undiagnosed COPD. Thus, in all, COPD probably affects 30 to 35 million people in the U.S. Accordingly, it is incumbent upon all primary care physicians to be alert to the possibility of COPD in patients with productive cough, particularly in those who suffer exercise-related dyspnea and have a family history of the disease, and definitely in those who are smokers. COPD must be identified early by simple spirometric measurement as discussed in Section F. ■

References

Health, United States, 1999. U.S. Department of Health and Human Services, Centers for Disease Control and Prevention. 1999 DHHS Publication #99-1232 pp179-180. Mortality statistics related to COPD.

Higgins M. Risk factors associated with chronic obstructive lung disease. Ann NY Acad Sci 1991;642:7-17. This is a recent review of all of the known risk factors for COPD.

Janoff A. Elastase and emphysema: Current assessment of the protease-antiprotease hypothesis. Am Rev Respir Dis 1985;132:417-433. A state-of-the-art review of the elastase mechanisms involved in the pathogenesis of emphysema and COPD.

Peto R, Speizer FE, Cochrane AL, et al. The relevance in adults of airflow obstruction, but not of mucus hypersecretion, to morbidity from chronic lung disease. Am Rev Respir Dis 1983;128:491-500. A classic article discussing the favorable effect of stopping smoking on the rate of decline in FEV_1 and on survival during a 20-year follow-up.

Petty TL. Chronic obstructive lung disease and other conditions of the chest. Chapter 55 in Matzen RN, Lang RL (eds). *Clinical Preventive Medicine*. St. Louis: CV Mosby, 1993. A complete review on methods for preventing premature morbidity and mortality in COPD and related disorders.

D. Pathogenesis

The term COPD refers to the clinical and physiological consequences of an amalgam of chronic respiratory diseases that nearly always includes varying degrees of emphysema and chronic obstructive bronchitis. Because airway hyperreactivity commonly accompanies COPD, asthma or asthmatic bronchitis may also contribute to the evolving pathological features. The generic definition of COPD includes the late sequelae of cystic fibrosis, diffuse bronchiectasis, rheumatoid bronchiolitis, and other unusual diseases. But the great majority of patients with COPD–those who are the subject of this book–are tobacco smokers who appear to differ from other smokers in their unusual susceptibility to tobacco smoke.

The mechanisms that underlie this susceptibility are largely unknown. Only one factor, alpha-1-antitrypsin deficiency, has been clearly identified, but it accounts for only a small fraction of all COPD cases. Exposure to environmental or occupational dusts and gases may also lead to COPD, and this exposure is believed to cause many cases not attributable to tobacco smoke, especially in developing countries. This discussion of the pathogenesis of COPD therefore includes a description of alpha-1-antitrypsin deficiency, the mechanisms by which tobacco smoke and other inhaled pollutants may cause emphysema and chronic obstructive bronchitis, and how these diseases culminate in chronic airflow obstruction. The pathogenic pathways for these conditions are not well understood, but they are probably linked to chronic inflammation of the lung parenchyma and airways.

Alpha-1-Antitrypsin Deficiency

An important discovery was announced in 1963 by Laurell and Eriksson, who reported that persons with a hereditary deficiency of alpha-1-antitrypsin (AAT), a powerful protease enzyme inhibitor, developed panlobular emphysema at a much earlier age than those with ordinary COPD. The circulating level of alpha-1-antitrypsin is genetically determined by a single gene on chromosome 14, and the serum protease inhibitor phenotype (Pi type) is governed by independent expression of the two parental alleles. Further investigation disclosed that nearly all (95%), of those persons afflicted with AAT deficiency are homozygous for the Z allele, and thus are designated Pi ZZ. Most healthy persons with normal levels of alpha-1-antitrypsin have M alleles and are designated Pi MM. Pi MZ persons have serum levels of alpha-1-antitrypsin that are intermediate between Pi MM and Pi ZZ phenotypes, but heterozygotes are not at increased risk for emphysema. Many other phenotypes have been described, but most are not associated with emphysema.

Alpha-1-antitrypsin can inhibit the activity of several proteolytic enzymes, particularly neutrophil elastase. It plays a key role in preventing tissue destruction from excessive proteolysis during inflammatory reactions. Most persons have sufficient alpha-1-antitrypsin in their lungs and bloodstream to protect the lungs from proteolytic enzyme-induced damage during inflammation caused by tobacco smoke, other inhaled toxins, or infections. In contrast, patients with Pi ZZ phenotypes who lack alpha-1-antitrypsin are unable to control these inflammatory reactions, and emphysema develops after unrestrained proteolysis has damaged the elastic fiber network and the extracellular matrix of the lungs.

Emphysema

The discovery that patients with extremely low levels of serum alpha-1-antitrypsin had clinical emphysema, coupled with the experimental observation that papain, a plant enzyme with elastinolytic properties, could induce emphysema when instilled into the lungs of laboratory animals, led to the elastase-antielastase hypothesis of the pathogenesis of emphysema. In its simplest form, the elastase-antielastase theory avers that the net balance between the elastinolytic activities unleashed by the neutrophilic component of inflammation and the antielastinolytic defenses of the lungs determines whether or not emphysema will develop. The balance is clearly tipped in favor of neutrophil elastase-induced damage in patients with Pi ZZ alpha-1-antitrypsin deficiency. Conceivably, the balance could be tipped in the same direction in tobacco smokers in whom exuberant inflammatory reactions release abundant neutrophil elastase and overwhelm normal antielastinolytic defenses. This argument was strengthened by the observation that activated neutrophils also release potent free radicals of oxygen that are capable of inactivating alpha-1-antitrypsin through oxidation even when AAT is present in normal amounts, thereby allowing unimpeded action of neutrophil elastase.

But this hypothesis, which was enthusiastically greeted some 30 years ago, is now considered a naive oversimplification of the complex processes at work. Clearly, other cells besides neutrophils, particularly macrophages and possibly mesenchymal cells, contribute to the development of emphysema. Also, many other enzymes besides neutrophil elastase (such as cathepsins G, B, L, and D, collagenase, gelatinase, and proteinase-3) participate in the destructive process. The concept is emerging that smoking and many other kinds of inflammatory injuries yield a cocktail of proteinases that destroy lung tissue in a coordinated action that culminates in emphysema. Thus, emphysema has been viewed as the lungs' stereotyped response to a variety of injurious insults.

Even if we accept this revised hypothesis, a fundamental question still remains: Why are only a small fraction of smokers (perhaps 15% to 20%) susceptible to the development of progressive airflow obstruction with emphysema? This profound question of "host variation" suggests that other unknown and important factors, either inherited or acquired, affect pathogenesis.

Chronic Obstructive Bronchitis

As stated, pulmonary emphysema nearly always coexists with some degree of chronic obstructive bronchitis with inflammation of both large and small airways. However, there are even more problems with chronic bronchitis than with emphysema in identifying the responsible pathogenic mechanisms, because neither the symptoms that define the syndrome of chronic bronchitis (chronic cough and sputum production) nor the pathological findings (inflammation and hyperplasia of the secretory structures) are specific for the disorder.

The kind of chronic obstructive bronchitis that we are concerned about is presumed to result from injury to the peripheral airways by tobacco smoke or environmental or occupational dusts and gases. These toxins undoubtedly behave like other injurious agents in that the severity of the resulting damage depends on the concentration of the inhalant and the duration of exposure. Thus, heavy and prolonged exposure, usually to cigarette smoke, is nearly always identifiable in patients with COPD.

Although the pathogenesis of tobacco-induced chronic bronchitis is incompletely understood, we do know that the repeated inhalation of tobacco smoke causes hyperplasia of mucous glands in the bronchi and an increase in the number and proportion of secretory cells in bronchioles, where a neutrophilic and mononuclear cell inflammatory reaction also occurs. Finding elastase in the sputum of patients with chronic bronchitis supports the suggestion that the antiproteolytic defenses are overwhelmed in this disorder, and that a proteolytic cascade, not unlike that which leads to emphysema, injures small airways and contributes to their narrowing. Nevertheless, it is again necessary to evoke "host factors" to account for differences in damage among smokers from what appears to be quantitatively similar exposure. We have almost no understanding about why some persons with chronic bronchitis relentlessly progress to severe airflow obstruction, while many others remain relatively stable despite the fact that they continue to smoke.

Chronic Airflow Obstruction

Twenty years ago it was thought that expiratory airflow obstruction could occur in only two ways: narrowing of airways, which was equated with chronic bronchitis, and loss of elastic recoil, which was associated with emphysema. Now, as recently emphasized by Thurlbeck, it is more reasonable to consider that tobacco smoke has a generalized injurious effect on the lungs and airways, and that expiratory airflow limitation is the consequence of multiple processes that may occur separately, but usually occur together in various combinations.

One injury leads to chronic bronchitis, one of the early effects of smoking on the central airways that has little effect on airflow. Another abnormality is bronchiolar inflammation, which narrows and deforms peripheral airways and is an important cause of airflow obstruction. A third is inflammation of the parenchyma, which causes emphysema and airflow obstruction by decreasing elastic recoil through damage to the lungs' connective tissue matrix. Finally, smoking-induced parenchymal inflammation and breakdown result when the attachments between alveolar walls and neighboring bronchioles are destroyed, allowing the airways to narrow because of a loss of tethering. ■

References

Laurell CB, Eriksson S. The electrophoretic alpha1-globulin pattern of serum in alpha1-antitrypsin deficiency. Scand J Lab Clin Med 1963;15:132-140. The original report on the association between alpha-1-antitrypsin and emphysema; still worth reading.

Snider GL, Faling LJ, Rennard SI. Chronic bronchitis and emphysema. in Murray JF, Nadel JA (eds), *Textbook of Respiratory Medicine,* 2nd ed. Philadelphia: WB Saunders, 1994, pp 1331-1397. An excellent comprehensive summary of the pathogenesis, diagnosis, and treatment of COPD.

Tetley TD. New perspectives on basic mechanisms in lung disease. 6. Protease imbalance: Its role in lung disease. Thorax 1993;48:560-565. A recent review of the elastase-antielastase hypothesis that stresses the multiplicity and complexity of the factors involved.

Thurlbeck WM. Emphysema then and now. Can Respir J 1994;1:21-39. The newest and best review of the pathology and pathologic-radiographic-clinical correlations of COPD.

E. Natural History

Given the lack of precise knowledge about the pathogenesis of emphysema and the anatomic derangements that lead to chronic airflow obstruction, many details about the natural history of COPD are poorly understood. There is, however, considerable information about the effects of smoking and smoking cessation on lung function, particularly as reflected by changes in expiratory flow rates. Additional data document that exposure to some environmental or occupational dusts and gases, including air pollution, act separately and worsen the damage done by smoking. Also, airway hyperreactivity may affect the natural history of smoking-induced airflow obstruction.

Two things are certain: First, the processes that culminate in the clinical disorder we call COPD are slow to evolve. With the exception of patients with alpha-1-antitrypsin deficiency, who may develop symptoms of respiratory impairment in middle age, most tobacco smokers are free of complaints except chronic cough and sputum production while the disorder is progressing, usually over decades. Second, there is considerable individual variation in the clinical consequences of similar smoking histories.
In fact, only about 15% to 20% of smokers develop clinically severe COPD.

Tobacco Smoking

Beginning at about 25 years of age, lung function in perfectly healthy persons starts to decline, usually along a slowly accelerating curvilinear path. Serial assessments of expiratory flow rates (measured as forced expiratory volume in one second, or FEV_1), show a decrease of about 20 to 30 ml per year. In contrast, numerous studies have shown that in tobacco smokers these FEV_1 values worsen at an increased rate. Moreover, heavy smokers tend to lose FEV_1 faster than light smokers, indicating that there is a rough dose-response in the magnitude of deterioration. There are those persons who are unusually susceptible to the effects of tobacco smoke and who lose FEV_1 at a greatly increased rate compared with other smokers. These concepts have

Figure 4 A Model of the Natural History of COPD

The natural history of COPD and the effects of smoking and smoking cessation. Adapted from Fletcher C, Peto R. B Med J 1977;1:1645-1648.

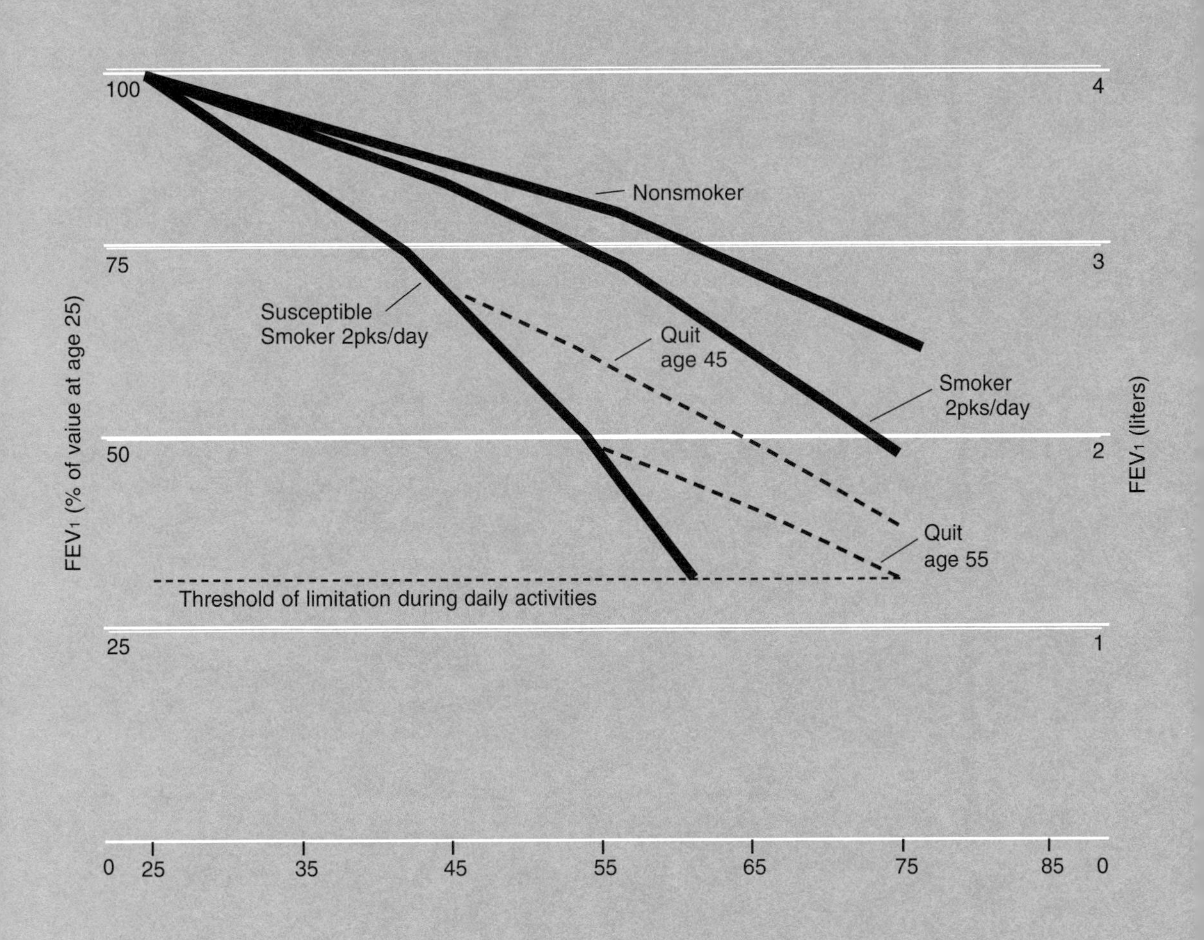

Table 1 The Lung Health Study: Deaths Within Five Years

Cause	Smoking Intervention and Ipratropium	Smoking Intervention and Placebo	Usual Care	Total
Lung Cancer	18	20	19	**57**
Cardiovascular Disease	18	7	12	**37**
Other	18	17	20	**55**
Total	**54**	**44**	**51**	**149**

Source: Anthonisen NR, et al

been incorporated into a model of the natural history of COPD, which was first proposed by Fletcher and Peto in 1977 and which has been updated in Figure 4. The benefits of smoking cessation are also shown.

In addition to the FEV_1, the forced vital capacity (FVC), and the ratio between these two (FEV_1/FVC), provide important information on the progress of disease. In fact, an association between the initial FEV_1 or FEV_1/FVC and the rate of subsequent deterioration in FEV_1 has been noted, particularly for men. Thus, a single number (an FEV_1/FVC lower than 70%), indicates the high likelihood that a patient is at risk of developing clinical COPD. So it is now possible to identify from among all middle-aged smokers those who are likely to develop disabling COPD as they grow older. This prediction becomes even stronger if serial studies over several years show an excessive rate of decline of FEV_1.

These observations formed the basis for the Lung Health Study, a five-year multicenter evaluation of the effects of early detection and intervention of COPD. This study, supported by the National Heart, Lung, and Blood Institute's Division of Lung Diseases, has already yielded much useful information. A late follow-up including 10-year observations on the cause of death is now underway. Thus far, the most common cause of death is lung cancer (See Table 1).

Recent studies have shown the expected inverse relationship between FEV_1 and pack-years of cigarettes smoked in COPD patients. The relationship between high smoking and low FEV_1 also correlates with increased neutrophils and IL-6, IL-8, and TNF alpha, which in turn, correlate with the percentage of neutrophils in the BAL. In addition, potentially pathogenic microbes are commonly found in the airways of smoking patients with high neutrophils and inflammatory cytokines, suggesting that they participate in a chronic inflammatory process, result in damage of alveoli and airways. The presence of high neutrophils and inflammatory cytokines is entirely compatible with the elastase imbalance theory and oxidant-induced injury theory of the pathogenesis of COPD.

Smoking Cessation

Virtually every study on the effects of smoking cessation has shown that it has clinical and physiologic benefits for both men and woman. In general, after cessation the exaggerated decline of FEV_1 noted in smokers gradually becomes similar to that found in nonsmokers, but the degree of initial improvement depends on the patient's age and type of respiratory impairment at the time of quitting. Smoking tobacco for 10 or more years causes airway inflammation in many persons, which is often accompanied by mild baseline bronchoconstriction and increased airway hyperreactivity. Because these abnormalities are inherently reversible, smokers who quit at this stage are likely to experience some initial improvement in their FEV_1 values as well as a reduced rate of decline in FEV_1 in subsequent years. In contrast, after 20 or more years of smoking-induced damage, the abnormalities become permanent and include emphysematous destruction of the lung parenchyma and chronic inflammation and distortion in the peripheral airways. Although stopping smoking at this time is beneficial in that it slows the rate of subsequent decline in FEV_1, the lack of reversibility in the lesions means that there is no short-term gain in pulmonary function. The latter concept is illustrated in Figure4, which shows that a susceptible continuing smoker will develop activity-restricting symptoms of COPD at about 62 years of age, but that if he or she stops smoking at 55 years of age, the onset of symptoms is delayed 12 years.

Occupational Dusts and Gases

The evidence is now persuasive that occupational dusts and gases cause an accelerated decline in FEV_1 in nonsmokers and, because these toxins interact with the effects of tobacco smoke, they cause an even greater decline in smokers. These effects have been well documented in workers exposed to mineral dusts and grain dusts, and result from other kinds of industrial exposures as well.

Air Pollution

Most studies of the long-term effects of chronic injury on pulmonary function have concentrated on tobacco smokers. Recently, however, data were published that reinforce observations that heavy environmental air pollution has a deleterious effect on FEV_1. This effect, like that from occupational dusts and gases, is apparent in nonsmokers and is clearly additive to the effects of smoking. Thus, the impact of chronic residential exposure to high levels of ambient air pollution may account for some of the COPD that develops in patients who have no significant exposure to tobacco smoke. In developing countries, indoor air pollution from cooking and heating sources is also believed to be an important cause of COPD.

Airway Hyperreactivity

Nonspecific airway hyperreactivity has been suggested as one of the "host factors" that predispose some tobacco smokers to the development of COPD. This hypothesis was recently supported by findings from the Lung Health Study. In 5,877 current smokers with early COPD who were tested with methacholine, 68.6% demonstrated airway hyperresponsiveness. Interestingly, the abnormality was more frequent in women (85.1%), than in men (58.9%), and could not be attributed to age, tobacco use, diagnosis of asthma, or baseline degree of airflow obstruction. Nevertheless, a pathogenic link between the presence of airway hyperreactivity and progressive COPD has not been conclusively established for two reasons. First, it is possible that both airway hyperresponsiveness and worsening airflow obstruction are separate outcomes of smoking that are not causally related. Second, it is possible that the airflow obstruction precedes the hyperreactivity, not the other way around (which is essential for the hypothesis to be correct). ■

References

Becklake MR. Occupational exposures: Evidence for a causal association with chronic obstructive pulmonary disease. Am Rev Respir Dis 1989;140:S85-S91. An excellent review with convincing evidence.

Fletcher C, Peto R. The natural history of chronic airflow obstruction. B Med J 1977;1:1645-1648. The classic and still one of the best studies on the subject.

Sherrill DL, Holberg CJ, Enright PL, et al. Longitudinal analysis of the effects of smoking onset and cessation on pulmonary function. Am J Respir Crit Care Med 1994;149:591-597. A good review of the subject.

Soler N, Ewig S, Torres A, et al. Airway inflammation and bronchial microbial patterns in patients with stable chronic obstructive pulmonary disease. Eur Respir J 1999;14:1015-1022. New research that implicates chronic microbial infestation or inflammation in activity neutrophils to release inflammatory cytokines that cause damage to airways and alveoli.

Tashkin DP, Altose MD, Bleecker ER, et al. The Lung Health Study: Airway responsiveness to inhaled methacholine in smokers with mild to moderate airflow limitation. Am Rev Respir Dis 1992;145:301-310. One of the largest and probably the best study of airway hyperresponsiveness in early COPD.

Tashkin DP, Detels R, Simmons M, et al. The UCLA population studies of chronic obstructive respiratory disease: XI. Impact of air pollution and smoking on annual change in forced expiratory volume in one second. Am J Respir Crit Care Med 1994;149:1209-1217. Persuasive evidence that ambient air pollution is hazardous.

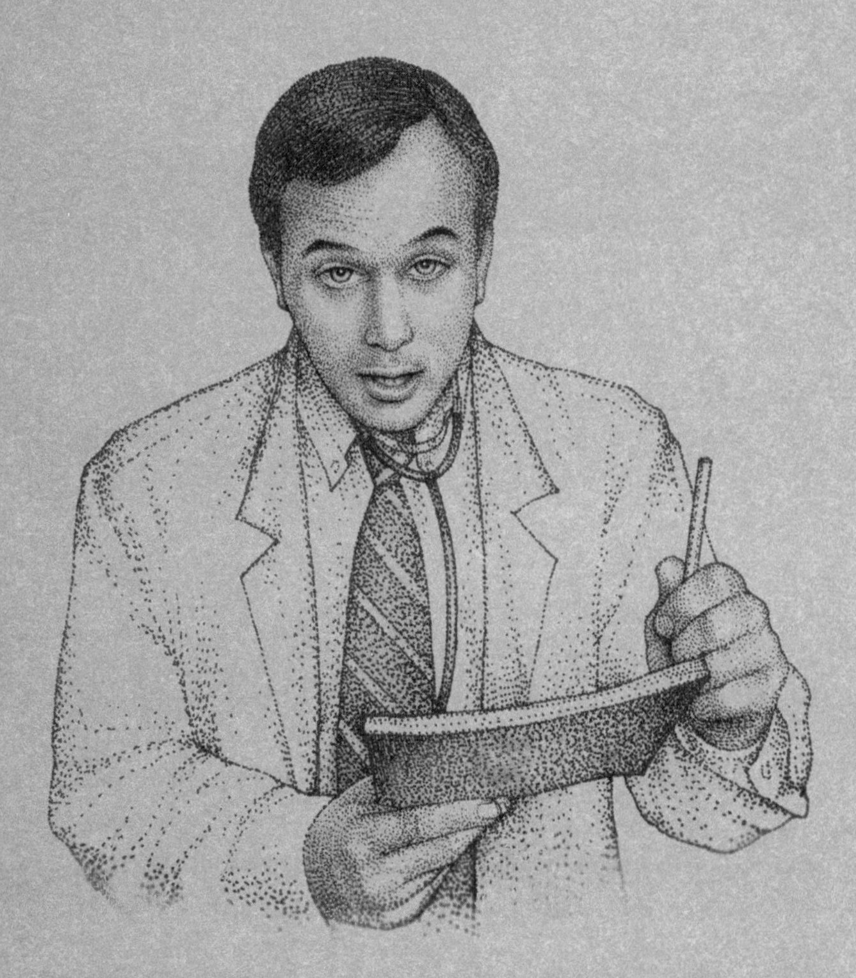

The primary care physician is in an ideal position to recognize COPD at its earliest stages, even before symptoms are present.

F. Diagnosis

The diagnosis of COPD is based on clinical criteria. The clinician arrives at a diagnosis only after careful consideration of the patient's history and physical examination, radiographic studies, pulmonary function studies, and certain laboratory tests. There is a recent justifiable emphasis on diagnosing COPD in its early, often asymptomatic stages by demonstrating abnormal FEV_1 values. Early intervention, especially smoking cessation, will improve pulmonary function or at least greatly slow the progress of airways obstruction. **This disease should not be allowed to progress to its final stages before it is recognized and treated.**

The primary care physician is in an ideal position to recognize COPD at its earliest stages, even before symptoms are present. Smokers should be screened systematically for airflow reduction by spirometry in the physician's office, just as other patients are screened for illnesses such as hypertension, hyperlipidemia, breast cancer, and uterine cancer.

Spirometry is the key test, but a questionnaire can also be helpful in screening for COPD and should be part of every patient's chart. Important items of information include:

1. Family History: Note history of allergies, emphysema, cystic fibrosis, COPD, and other chronic lung conditions.
2. Smoking History: Indicate age of smoking initiation and number of packs smoked per day.
3. Detailed Occupational History: Detail any exposure to noxious inhalants.
4. History of Respiratory Tract Infections: Note frequency and severity.
5. Current Symptoms: Document dyspnea, cough, wheezing, sputum production, and chest pain.

(continued)

There are many standardized forms available to the physician for documenting the pulmonary history. A sample form is found in Appendix A.

The most common presenting complaint in a patient with COPD is dyspnea on exertion, a symptom that develops late in the course of this disease. The patient may not acknowledge the classic early symptoms: morning cough and sputum production. A history of recurrent respiratory tract infections, which are usually prolonged and often require antibiotic treatment, is common. A childhood history of frequent respiratory tract infections and bronchitis may indicate the presence of asthma at an early age. Any history of typical asthma, recurrent sinus infections, or nasal polyps should be noted, because such conditions are common in patients with COPD. A smoking history is, obviously, of paramount importance.

Complaints of dyspnea, cough, and sputum production may be associated with a number of other pulmonary and nonpulmonary problems. The primary care physician should exclude other conditions such as neoplasm, cardiac failure, infection, inflammatory disease, and genetic and hypersensitivity diseases. These, of course, may coexist with COPD.

The patient's physical examination is likely to be entirely normal early in the course of COPD. However, decreased breath sounds, wheezes, and crackles at the bases might be observed, especially during exacerbations. Pursed-lip breathing, intercostal retractions, edema, cyanosis, and evidence of weight loss are seen only with advanced disease.

Radiographic Studies

Both posteroanterior and lateral chest x-rays are required in the evaluation of COPD, but they are of no value as screening tools. Chest x-rays are useful in ruling out other causes of respiratory symptoms. The finding of apparently hyperlucent lungs has frequently led to the false diagnosis of airways obstruction. X-rays can show low, flat diaphragms, enlarged retrosternal air space, sparse vasculature in the periphery of the lung fields, bullous lesions, and pulmonary artery prominence, but these develop only in the later stages of COPD.

Computerized tomography, (CT), scans are rarely indicated, but the use of high-resolution, thin-cut CT images is currently being evaluated in the diagnosis of interstitial lung disease. The technique may prove to be of value in assessing the early stages of COPD in selected patients. CT is also helpful in the early diagnosis of COPD, where the risk of lung cancer is high.

Electrocardiogram

The electrocardiogram is normal in the early stages of COPD, but peaked P-waves in II, III, AVF, decreased voltage of QRS, and right axis deviation are often noted in advanced stages of disease. Supraventricular arrhythmias are commonly found as well, especially during exacerbations.

Laboratory Screening

Testing in the clinical laboratory is rarely useful in the diagnosis of COPD. Patients with a family history of severe, early-onset emphysema, however, should be screened for alpha-1-antitrypsin deficiency. Also, secondary erythrocytosis may reflect chronic hypoxemia, a late manifestation.

(continued)

Spirometry

A spirometer used for screening purposes must be available to the primary care physician in the office setting. Spirometry is used to identify patients with COPD by measuring their expiratory flow rates and vital capacity. It may be used to assess the severity of a patient's disease. Serial tests allow the physician to measure the patient's response to therapy. The use of spirometry has also been shown to be a useful tool in motivating patients to stop smoking.

There is little to support routine screening in the general population. But smokers and other patients exposed to injurious inhalants should be routinely screened. All patients who complain of dyspnea or unexplained cough should receive pulmonary function tests.

The forced vital capacity (FVC), the forced expiratory volume in one second (FEV_1), and the ratio of these two (FEV_1/FVC), are the primary spirometric measurements used for diagnosis. A reduced FEV_1/FVC (less than 70%), indicates airways obstruction. The severity of airflow obstruction is also reflected in the FEV_1. A reduced FVC may suggest restrictive dysfunction, but this cannot be determined reliably by spirometry alone.

As discussed in Section M, the National Lung Health Education Program, (NLHEP), the FEV_6 is used as a surrogate marker for FVC. The advantage is more convenience in clinical spirometric testing. The FEV_1/FEV_6 ratio tracks the classic FEV_1/FVC ratio quite accurately, and identifies patients at risk of rapid declines in FEV_1 over time.

Repeating spirometric tests after administering an inhaled bronchodilator to patients may help identify a bronchospastic element of their disease. An improvement in the FVC or FEV_1 of 15% or more, according to American Thoracic Society standards, indicates a positive response. Failure to respond does not necessarily mean that a patient will not find bronchodilators or corticosteroids helpful.

Many manufacturers sell spirometers that give rapid results. Many are computerized and their use requires little training. All equipment should meet the American Thoracic Society's performance recommendations and should be calibrated regularly to assure continued accuracy. It is strongly recommended that physicians use a spirometer that produces a hard copy of the flow-volume loop and/or the time-volume curve for inclusion in the patient's chart.

Other Pulmonary Function Tests

Complete pulmonary function studies are not necessary in the routine evaluation of early COPD. Indications for referral to the pulmonary function laboratory include:

1. The evaluation of dyspnea of uncertain etiology.
2. Disability evaluation.
3. Preoperative evaluation of a patient requiring thoracic or intra-abdominal surgery.

Specific tests can help in the diagnosis and treatment of conditions related to COPD. Hyperinflation is manifested in COPD by an increase in total lung capacity and an increase in the ratio of residual volume to total lung volume capacity. Emphysema or interstitial lung disease is suggested by a reduction in the diffusing capacity. The use of pulse oximetry to estimate oxygen saturation is useful, but arterial blood gas measurements are necessary to assess and manage patients during exacerbations and when oxygen therapy is prescribed. ■

References

American Thoracic Society. Lung function testing, selection of reference values, and interpretation strategies. Am Rev Resp Dis 1991;144:1202-1218. An excellent source of useful information.

American Thoracic Society. Standards for the diagnosis and care of patients with chronic obstructive pulmonary disease (COPD) and asthma. An official statement of the American Thoracic Society. Am Rev Respir Dis 1987;136:225-245. This is a well-referenced six-chapter review on useful approaches to the diagnosis of COPD and associated asthma.

Crapo RO. Current concepts: Pulmonary function testing. N Engl J Med 1994;331:25-30. All the primary care physician needs to know about pulmonary function testing.

Ferguson GT, Enright PL, Buist AS, Higgins MW. Office spirometry for lung health assessment in adults. A consensus statement from the National Lung Health Education Program, (NLHEP). Chest 2000;117:1146-1161. This consensus statement from the NLHEP recommends spirometric testing for all smokers over age 45 and anyone with dyspnea, cough, mucus, or wheeze.

Hankinson JL, Odencrantz JR, Fedan KB. Spirometric reference values from a sample of the general U.S. population. Am J Respir Crit Care Med 1999;159:179-187. An update review of spirometric reference values from a large randomized sample of the United States population. The FEV_6 is a good surrogate marker of FVC and the FEV_1/FEV_6 ratio is useful in identifying subjects with rapid rates of decline in FEV.

Management
Stable COPD

The careful management of COPD in the outpatient setting can effectively improve symptoms, minimize deterioration in pulmonary function, and prevent hospitalization during acute exacerbations. There are four phases in the primary care physician's strategy to meet these goals:

1. Stress smoking cessation and patient education about the disease.
2. Improve pulmonary function as much as possible by treating any reversible component of the patient's lung disease and by establishing a therapeutic "plateau" to prevent accelerated deterioration in pulmonary function as the patient grows older.
3. Treat acute exacerbations of COPD in the outpatient setting.
4. Prevent non-COPD complications of therapy.

ase 1

Smoking Cessation and Patient Education

The primary care physician is in an ideal position to emphasize the importance of smoking cessation to all patients, but especially those with early or moderately advanced COPD. Educate your patients about the damaging effect of tobacco smoke on the progression of the disease process and on the worsening of their pulmonary function. Explain to patients that when they stop smoking they will reap many benefits, including reduced airway secretions, reduced airway inflammation, and reduced bronchospasm.

It helps to discuss the importance of behavior modification and smoking addiction. Frequently, a patient is receptive to their physician's recommendation about a nicotine patch or referral to a smoking cessation class. It is important to schedule follow-up visits in the clinic to reinforce the patient's decision to quit smoking (See Section J).

(continued)

In addition, educating the patient and his or her family about COPD, the importance of complying with medication regimens, and the value of exercise is vital to the successful management of the disease.

The most useful approach to smoking cessation is counseling that quitting is absolutely essential. Picking a quit date is key to the entire process. A variety of pharmacologic agents are available to mitigate nicotine withdrawal symptoms. These are summarized in Table 2.

When nicotine replacement is chosen, it should be started on the quit date. The advantage of the gum is that it allows the patient to titrate the rate of nicotine absorption. Four mg gum is more effective than 2 mg gum in patients who are most heavily addicted, i.e., smoking more than one pack a day, and beginning early in the morning, with the morning cigarette being the most important. When bupropion is given, it should be initiated approximately one week before the quit date. The nicotine products can be used in combination. Even if used together in full manufacturers' doses, it is unlikely that nicotine blood levels will exceed those produced regularly by the addicted smoker. A combination of nicotine replacement and bupropion has resulted in the highest success in biologically proven cessation one year after initiation of therapy.

(continued)

Table 2 Drugs Used for Smoking Cessation

Drug and Method of Administration	Unit Dose	Dose Interval
Nicotine polacrilex (oral)	2 to 4 mg	Every 1 to 2 hours*
Transdermal nicotine patch	21, 14, and 7 mg 15, 10, and 5 mg 22 and 11 mg	Over 24 hours Over 16 hours Over 24 hours
Nasal nicotine spray	0.5 mg/inhalation/nostril	8 to 40 mg/day in hourly or p.r.n. dosing
Nicotine inhaler	10 mg/inhaler	Inhale for 20 minutes 6 to 16 times/day
Bupropion sustained-release tablets	150 mg	150 mg for 3 days, then 300 mg/day
Buspirone tablets	15, 10, and 5 mg	7.5 mg b.i.d., starting dose; 60 mg/day, maximum dose

* Fifteen to 30 pieces may be chewed over 24 hours.

References

Hankinson JL, Odencrantz JR, Fedan KB. Spirometric reference values from a sample of the general U.S. population. Am J Respir Crit Care Med 1999;159:179-187. An updated review. The FEV_6 is a good surrogate marker of FVC and the FEV_1/FEV_6 ratio is useful in identifying subjects with rapid rates of decline in FEV.

Hilleman DE, Mohiuddin SM, Del Core MG, Sketch MH Sr. Effect of buspirone on withdrawal symptoms associated with smoking cessation. Arch Intern Med 1992;152:350-352. This non-benzodiazepine was effective in reducing the symptoms of nicotine withdrawal.

Hurt RD, Dale LC, Fredrickson PA, et al. Nicotine patch therapy for smoking cessation combined with physician advice and nurse follow-up. One-year outcome and percentage of nicotine replacement. JAMA 1994;271:595-600. This randomized trial showed that the nicotine patch increased smoking cessation more than physician advice and nurse follow-up.

Hurt RD, Sachs DP, Glover ED, et al. A comparison of sustained-release bupropion and placebo for smoking cessation. N Engl J Med 1997;337:1195-1202. This randomized clinical trail demonstrated the effectiveness of bupropion compared with placebo.

Jorenby DE, Keehn DS, Fiore MC. Comparative efficacy and tolerability of nicotine replacement therapies. CNS Drugs. 1995;3:227-236. A review of the effectiveness of drugs used in nicotine withdrawal.

Jorenby DE, Leischow SJ, Nides MA, et al. A controlled trial of sustained-release bupropion, a nicotine patch, or both for smoking cessation. N Engl J Med 1999; 340:685-691. A greater quit rate was achieved with combined therapy compared with either agent used separately.

Phase 2

Treating the Reversible Component of COPD and Establishing a Therapeutic Plateau

Early COPD

During the patient's initial visit, the physician should establish a "baseline" measurement of pulmonary function using information from the patient's history, physical examination, and spirometric test results. This is also the appropriate time to quickly rule out other factors that can exacerbate pulmonary symptoms, such as seasonal or allergic contributions. Questions about the "triggers" that cause dyspnea, wheezing, or cough, which might suggest "hidden asthma" presenting as COPD, are an important part of the history. It is usually not necessary to perform atopic skin testing or inhalation challenge tests to evaluate COPD.

Premature deterioration in lung function in patients without obvious asthma should prompt the physician to further investigate the possibility of protease-inhibitor deficiency by screening for alpha-1-antitrypsin deficiency. Other factors such as occupational exposure to particulate dusts, fumes, air pollution, or wood stoves may be important.

Other coexisting illnesses that may contribute to airflow obstruction include recurrent sinus infections, allergic rhinitis, chest infections, severe esophageal reflux, and an underlying illness such as congestive heart failure, liver disease, or malignancy. The presence of these conditions might affect decisions about medication.

Carefully review and eliminate any medication taken by the patient that may be contributing to cough or bronchospasm or causing an adverse drug interaction. These might include beta-blocking drugs, ACE inhibitors, diuretics, theophyllines, tranquilizers, and hypnotics. Theophylline interacts with many medications, all of which tend to increase theophylline levels. These include: cimetidine, fluconazole, and macrolide (e.g., erythromycin), and quinolone (e.g., ciprofloxacin) antibiotics. In patients of advanced age, or who have liver disease or congestive heart failure, the metabolism of theophylline is also delayed.

It is important to measure the patient's baseline pulmonary function using spirometry, both to support the diagnosis and to have a standard against which to measure the patient's response to treatment. This is especially true when the use of corticosteroids is considered, because patient education regarding the benefits and risks of this class of medications is very important.

Pulse oximetry can be used in the office when the patient is "at rest" and when "ambulating" to establish the presence of hypoxemia. This test can also disclose the problem of oxygen desaturation during simple activities of daily living, (ADLS), which so frequently prevents patients with COPD from engaging in simple exercise at home (See Sections F and I).

Medication Treatment

Bronchodilators

After the initial spirometric testing is complete, develop an individualized medication program for the patient that includes bronchodilators to improve airflow and to reduce dyspnea. The first medication tried should be ipratropium, delivered via a metered-dose inhaler, (MDI), with or without the concomitant use of an inhaled beta-adrenergic (e.g., albuterol, bitolterol, pirbuterol, meta-proterenol, salmeterol), also delivered via an MDI. It is essential to thoroughly demonstrate the correct technique for using the MDI as outlined in Table 3 and illustrated in Figure 5. Patients with poor coordination who cannot master the press-and-breathe technique may need to use a spacer or a breath-activated device, which should allow nearly all patients to use MDI's correctly. A common mistake is to prescribe these effective medications without adequate patient instruction or follow-up to monitor their use, the patient's response to treatment, and any objective improvement in airflow.

Ipratropium bromide and albuterol sulfate are now available in a single inhaler marketed as Combivent® Inhalation Aerosol. Several studies have shown that the combination is more effective than either agent used alone. Combivent® Inhalation Aerosol is used for maintenance treatment but can also be used to manage breakthrough attacks. Thus, it is one of the most versatile agents to use in COPD. The combination product may improve compliance and reduce cost.

If necessary, add either theophylline (200 to 300 mg b.i.d.) and/or slow release albuterol tablets (4 to 8 mg daily or b.i.d. if tolerated) when persistent dyspnea, lack of objective improvement, or "breakthrough" symptoms of cough, wheezing, or nocturnal exacerbations are present. Many patients cannot tolerate the tremor and gastrointestinal side effects that may accompany oral theophylline or albuterol preparations. Slow-release theophylline preparations give the best nocturnal blood levels and lessen gastrointestinal intolerance. Tremor, which may accompany the use of albuterol preparations, can be minimized by gradually increasing the dose over one or two weeks' time.

Consider adding the new long-acting beta-adrenergic, salmeterol (delivered via an MDI), to help control breakthrough symptoms or to improve medication compliance. Its benefit in asthma is its long duration (10 to 12 hours), but its role in COPD is not yet defined. Patients using this drug need to be reminded to continue using their other inhaled bronchodilators when needed for "rescue therapy," since salmeterol takes 75 to 90 minutes to begin acting.

(continued)

Table 3 How to Use an MDI

How to Use an MDI	Check how much medicine is in the canister.
	1. If the canister is new, it is full.
	2. If the canister has been used repeatedly, it might be empty. The product label should show how many inhalations should be in each canister.
	To check how much medicine is left in the canister, put the canister (not the mouthpiece) in a cup of water. If the canister sinks to the bottom, it is full. If the canister floats sideways on the surface, it is empty.
How to Use the Inhaler	**1.** Remove the cap and hold the inhaler upright.
	2. Shake the inhaler.
	3. Tilt your head back slightly and breathe out.
	4. Position the inhaler in one of the ways illustrated in Figure 5.
	5. Press down on the inhaler to release medication as you start to breathe in slowly.
	6. Breathe in slowly (3 to 5 seconds).
	7. Hold breath for 10 seconds to allow medicine to reach deeply into the lungs.
	8. Repeat puffs as directed. Waiting 1 minute between puffs may permit the second puff to penetrate the lungs better.
	9. Spacers are useful for all patients. They are particularly recommended for young children and older adults and for use with inhaled corticosteroids.

Figure 5 Proper Press-and-Breathe Techniques for MDI Use

A. Open mouth with inhaler 1 to 2 inches away

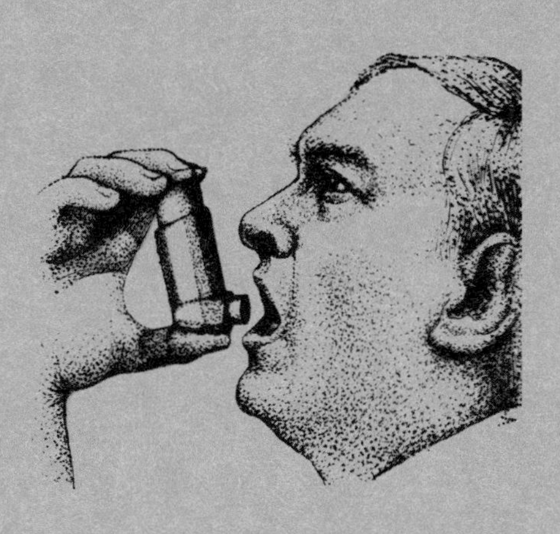

B. Use spacer

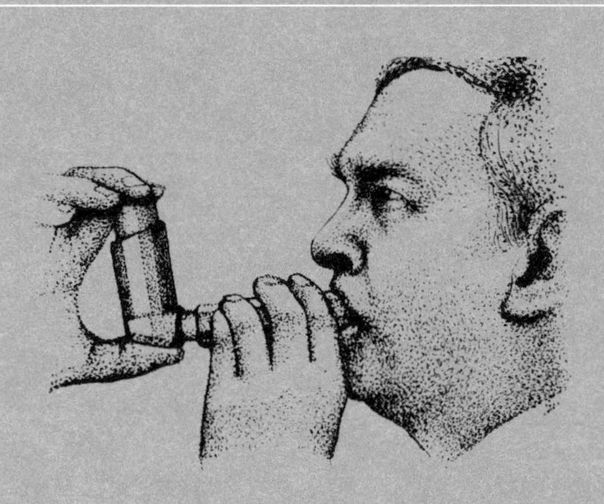

C. In the mouth for breath activated devices

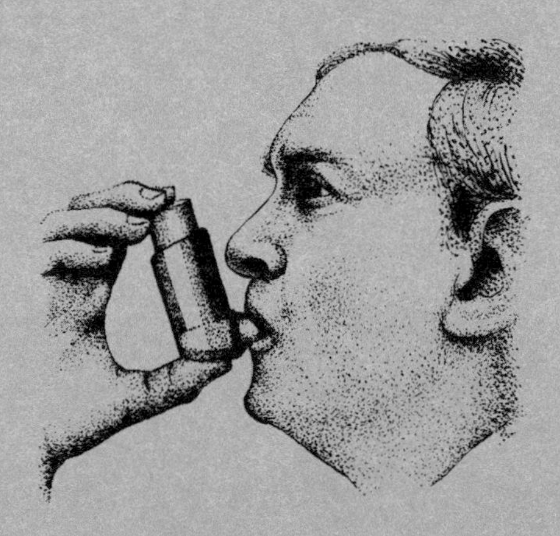

Corticosteroids

The use of corticosteroids in patients with COPD is controversial, but many patients benefit from short- or long-term use. The physician should clearly document in the patient record the rationale for using this therapy. Baseline measurements of spirometric data and objective assessments of the patient's response to treatment during follow-up visits should also be documented.

A trial of oral corticosteroids is indicated in patients with severe airflow limitation or in patients who continue to deteriorate despite maximal bronchodilator therapy. A typical course of steroids would be: Prednisone 40 to 60 mg daily for seven days, then gradually tapering over ten days to 10 to 20 mg daily or every other day, at which time the patient should be reassessed in the office objectively by spirometry and, if appropriate, oximetry.

Long-term corticosteroid use for patients with COPD should be maintained only in those who experience a documented improvement in their airflow obstruction after treatment. The lowest dose possible should be used and attention should be given to preventing potential side effects. The physician may want to taper the steroid to alternate-day use, adding an inhaled corticosteroid medication, to minimize systemic side effects.

Inhaled corticosteroids might also be considered for use along with inhaled bronchodilators to gain some of the therapeutic benefits of steroids while avoiding the systemic side effects associated with long-term oral steroid therapy. Four drugs are available: beclomethasone (2 to 4 puffs q.i.d.), flunisolide (2 to 4 puffs b.i.d.), fluticisone in three different strengths (2 puffs b.i.d.), and triamcinolone (2 to 4 puffs q.i.d.). Careful rinsing of the mouth after nebulization and the use of spacers will minimize oral moniliasis.

Nebulized bronchodilators

Patients with advanced COPD or those who have difficulty using a metered-dose inhaler, either routinely or during acute exacerbations, may benefit from the use of an "updraft" or "wet" nebulizer system of inhaled ipratropium (available as a unit dose medication) or beta-adrenergic bronchodilators. The beta-adrenergic medications available for routine outpatient use include: albuterol (unit dose vial .083 mg/ml, or 0.5 ml with 2 ml normal saline), metaproterenol (unit dose vial 0.6% or 0.4%, or 0.3 ml with 2 ml normal saline), terbutaline (unit dose vial), or bitolterol (0.75 to 1 ml). Ipratropium and a beta-adrenergic agent may be used together in an updraft nebulizer.

Mucolytic drugs

Consider adding a mucolytic agent (e.g., guaifenesin, 600 mg 1 to 4 times daily) if the patient has difficulty clearing secretions. Acetylcysteine may improve sputum clearance and loosen mucous plugs in patients with severe bronchitis, bronchiectasis, or cystic fibrosis, but because this drug may cause bronchospasm, it is usually administered in an updraft nebulizer with a bronchodilator.

(continued)

Advanced COPD

Patients with advanced COPD are typically treated with both oral and inhaled bronchodilators. Careful attention to the presence of underlying sinus and bronchial infections will help prevent further deterioration in pulmonary function (See Section H.1). Oxygen therapy, regular exercise, and corticosteroid therapy also frequently play an important role in the treatment of advanced COPD. Close follow-up in the outpatient setting, with regular monitoring of the patient's pulmonary function, oxygenation, and ambulatory ability are necessary to treat this challenging group of patients effectively.

The physician should regularly review the important aspects of the treatment program with the patient, including the pathophysiology of COPD, the pursed-lip breathing technique, the correct MDI technique, the importance of smoking cessation and exercise, and the necessity of compliance with medication regimens.

Oxygen Therapy

Frontline physicians should evaluate each patient's oxygenation using oximetry, and should consider prescribing continuous oxygen therapy for those who have resting room air saturations of less than 88% or ambulatory saturations of less than 88%. Clinical consideration must be given for exceptions to these specific guidelines, of course, but ongoing, untreated hypoxemia will accelerate the development of cor pulmonale, negatively affect cognitive function, increase respiratory muscle fatigue, reduce the quality of sleep, and diminish the patient's tolerance for mild exercise or even the simplest activities of daily living (See Sections H.5 and I). Primary care physicians may consider referring well-selected, motivated patients for transtracheal oxygen therapy which may improve comfort, reduce respiratory muscle fatigue, and improve mobility by reducing the oxygen flow rate required.

Ambulatory oxygen has become the standard of care for patients who can and will increase their exercise beyond the 50 feet of tubing that connects with a stationary source. The Nocturnal Oxygen Therapy Trial, (NOTT), showed a superiority of ambulatory oxygen with a superior survival from continuous oxygen therapy, (COT), provided from an ambulatory source, compared with nocturnal oxygen therapy, (NOT), provided by a stationary source. Of course, the duration of oxygen administration was greater with COT, (mean 17.7 hours, median 19.4 hours per day), compared with ambulatory oxygen, (11.8 hours per day). Thus, the improved survival could have been the result of the method or the duration of oxygen therapy. A re-analysis of the NOTT data strongly suggests that the ability to increase exercise along with the provision of ambulatory oxygen was the most likely reason for improved survival in the NOTT.

Phase 3

Treating Acute Exacerbations of COPD in the Outpatient Setting

During an acute exacerbation of COPD, the physician will need to increase inhaled bronchodilator frequency, possibly add an updraft nebulizer, treat underlying sinusitis or pulmonary infection (See Section H.1), and frequently add a course of corticosteroids to prevent further deterioration and to avoid hospitalization resulting from increasing bronchospasm, air trapping, respiratory muscle fatigue, and ultimately respiratory failure. Oxygen needs should be assessed and oral bronchodilator medication added or increased, if tolerated. Inhaled bronchodilators give the patient the most rapid relief from acute bronchospasm, and continuous nebulization of albuterol has been shown to be safe for status asthmaticus for 45 to 90 minutes.

Indications for emergent hospitalization include: acute respiratory failure manifested by either worsening hypoxemia or acute respiratory acidosis; clinical signs of marked fatigue secondary to the increased work of breathing and manifested by tachypnea (respiratory rate greater than 30 breaths per minute), tachycardia, and the vigorous use of accessory respiratory muscles; and/or pneumonia causing respiratory compromise or other medical complications.

Phase 4

Preventing Non-COPD Complications of Therapy

Patients using long-term corticosteroids or with reduced mobility or advancing age are at risk for compression fractures due to accelerated osteoporosis. A good anti-osteoporosis program should include: exercise (simple walking is best); corticosteroid dose reduced to as low as possible, substituting inhaled corticosteroids if effective; calcium supplements; estrogen supplements if appropriate (consider the use of progesterone if clinically indicated); and etidronate (400 mg q.d. for two weeks, every three months for two years) for patients who are unable to reduce their prednisone dose to less than 20 mg every other day or who are otherwise at high risk for osteoporosis.

Patients with COPD benefit from a good nasal hygiene program, especially if they use a nasal cannula for oxygen therapy. The use of nasal saline lavage, inhaled nasal corticosteroids, and increased humidification can help patients who experience increased nasal congestion. Decongestants containing pseudoephedrine and guaifenesin are well tolerated when topical measures do not control rhinorrhea or congestion.

Review the patient's medication list to see if any obvious drugs are contributing to their symptoms. Check the theophylline blood level (the goal is 8 to 12 μg/ml) if a patient is exhibiting clinical signs of toxicity (gastrointestinal symptoms, tremor, headache, tachycardia), or when adding another medication that may affect the metabolism of theophylline. Rule out possible metabolic side effects such as hyperglycemia, hypokalemia, or azotemia when a change in the patient's clinical condition occurs or when initiating corticosteroid or diuretic therapy.

Recognize and treat depression and marked anxiety, which frequently accompany COPD. It helps to discuss this openly with the patient and their family and consider a psychiatric referral when simple measures (counseling, improving exercise and sleep routines, and maximizing pulmonary function) do not help control the patient's symptoms. Patients with stable COPD tolerate antidepressant therapy quite well, but most often depression is relieved when their "airflow obstruction" and "anxiety" are treated. Consider the use of alprazolam (0.25 mg q6h) or lorazepam (0.5 mg to 1.0 mg q6h to 8h) in patients with disabling panic disorder that accompanies their COPD. Avoid overusing tranquilizer medications. They can affect mental acuity or cause excessive drowsiness. Encourage patients to avoid the regular use of hypnotic medications.

Conclusion

The earlier the diagnosis of COPD, the longer the preservation of lung function. This underscores the need for office spirometry to make an early diagnosis. The primary care physician can, through careful interest and perseverance, help patients with more advanced COPD deal with their chronic disability. An emphasis on smoking cessation, compliance with medication programs, exercise, and oxygen therapy when necessary will in most cases improve–and often stabilize–pulmonary function. Most often, patients will "plateau" and will experience long periods between "relapses" or exacerbations. These plateaus are very gratifying to patients, their families, and the physician and clinic staff.

When interviewing patients, look for certain symptoms (such as increased dyspnea, cough, fever, edema, or fatigue) that might suggest a nonspecific exacerbation of their COPD. The practitioner becomes very sensitive to changes in a patient's condition. Increased depression, fatigue, a change in sleep habits, decreased appetite, or other unexplained symptoms may in fact be the clinical manifestations of a deterioration in pulmonary function. A brief physical examination focusing on the work required by breathing and the appearance of the patient, brief spirometric recordings and oximetry readings, or a change on the patient's chest x-ray frequently give clues about the patient's clinical deterioration. These same details can suggest changes in the patient's medication program that might prevent hospitalization and further deterioration in pulmonary function. ■

References

Bone RC. A step-care approach to managing COPD. J Respir Dis 1991;12:727-740. A practical guide to the pharmacologic management of COPD.

Casaburi R, Petty TL (eds). *Principles and Practice of Pulmonary Rehabilitation.* Chicago: WB Saunders, 1993; 508 pages. A full-length textbook on pulmonary rehabilitation for COPD and related disorders such as asthma, cystic fibrosis, and interstitial lung disease.

Dorinsky PM, Reisner C, Ferguson GT, et al. The combination of ipratropium and albuterol optimizes pulmonary function reversibility testing in patients with COPD. Chest 1999;115:966-971. A greater increase in FEV_1 was found in 1,067 stable COPD patients, 30 minutes after inhaling the combination. This response exceeded the FEV responses from the individual drugs.

Ferguson GT, Cherniack RM. Management of chronic obstructive pulmonary disease. N Engl J Med 1993;328:1017-1022. A thorough review of all the treatment medications that are useful in the management of COPD.

Ikeda A, Nishimura K, Koyama H, Izumi T. Bronchodilating effects of combined therapy with clinical dosages of ipratropium bromide and salbutamol for stable COPD: Comparison with ipratropium alone. Chest 1995;107:401-405. Salmeterol is the name for albuterol outside of the U.S.A. This report showed an additive effect from salbutamol (albuterol) added to ipratropium.

Petty TL (Chairman). Combivent Inhalation Aerosol Study Group. In chronic obstructive pulmonary disease, a combination of ipratropium and albuterol is more effective than either agent alone. An 85-day multicenter trial. Chest 1994;105:1411-1419. The initial report on the increased peak effect and longer duration of the combination product compared with each component.

Petty TL (Chairman). Nocturnal Oxygen Therapy Trial Group, (NOTT). Continuous or nocturnal oxygen therapy in hypoxemic chronic obstructive lung disease. A clinical trial. Ann Intern Med 1980;93:391-398. This multicenter trial demonstrated improved survival with continuous oxygen therapy provided by an ambulatory system compared with nocturnal oxygen delivered from a stationary system.

Petty TL, Bliss PL. Ambulatory oxygen therapy, exercise, and survival with advanced COPD. Respir Care 2000;45:204-211. This retrospective analysis of survival and hospitalizations revealed that ability to increase exercise and receiving ambulatory oxygen resulted in better outcomes compared with patients who had less ability to exercise and who received oxygen from a stationary source.

Treatment Complications

H.1 Intercurrent Infections

While a variety of noninfectious irritants and allergens can cause acute exacerbations in the patient with COPD, the most frequent and important are the infectious complications. These are extremely variable and range from nonspecific bronchitis to life-threatening pneumonia. The most common infectious complications associated with COPD are:

1. Acute purulent bronchitis.
2. Recurrent chronic bronchitis and bronchiectasis.
3. Community-acquired pneumonia.
4. Mycobacterial and fungal infections.

Acute Purulent Bronchitis

Patients with COPD and acute bronchitis present with increased amounts of purulent secretions, dyspnea, and chest tightness. The organisms most often identified include pneumococcus, hemophilus, and streptococcus. These usually respond to standard "first-line" antibiotics such as amoxicillin, doxycycline, trimethoprim-sulfamethoxazole, or erythromycin. Not only are these antibiotics effective antimicrobials, but they are the most cost effective. The effectiveness of erythromycin against *H. influenzae* is variable. The newer macrolides, clarithromycin and azithromycin, are more effective against *H. influenzae* but are substantially more expensive. These macrolides are also better tolerated and cause fewer gastrointestinal side effects than erythromycin.

Some patients with long-standing COPD become infected with gram-negative organisms (e.g., *Klebsiella, Serratia,* and *Pseudomonas*). These require specific treatment with third-generation cephalosporins or quinolones (See Table 4).

(continued)

Table 4 Empiric Antibiotic Therapy for Acute Purulent Bronchitis

First-Line Treatment

First-Line Treatment	Dose*
amoxicillin	250 to 500 mg t.i.d.
trimethoprim, (TM)–sulfamethoxazole, (SM)	1 capsule b.i.d. (160 mg TM, 800 mg SM)
doxycycline	100 mg b.i.d.
erythromycin	250 to 500 mg q.i.d.

Second-Line Treatment

Second-Line Treatment	Dose*
second-generation cephalosporin (e.g., cefuroxime)	250 mg b.i.d. to 500 mg b.i.d.
third-generation cephalosporin (e.g., cefixime)	400 mg q.i.d.
macrolides:	
clarithromycin	250 to 500 mg b.i.d.
azithromycin	500 mg day 1, then 250 mg q.d. x 5 days
quinolones:	
ciprofloxacin	750 mg b.i.d.
levofloxacin	500 mg b.i.d.

The designation "first-line" implies the most cost-effective antibiotics. The selection of antibiotics must be patient specific."Second-line" antibiotics are used in cases of allergy to or failure of first-line drugs.

* Dosages assume normal renal and/or hepatic function.

Acute purulent bronchitis should be treated for 7 days. Symptoms usually improve after 3 to 4 days of therapy. Because of associated bronchospasm, the patient's bronchodilator and anti-inflammatory therapy should be maximized. Frequently, this requires the addition of systemic corticosteroids.

Chronic Bronchitis and Bronchiectasis

If the initial course of therapy with first-line antibiotics fails, then a second course with broad-spectrum antibiotics (such as second- or third-generation cephalosporins, amoxicillin clavulanate, macrolides or quinolones), should be given for an additional 10 days.

While patients with chronic bronchitis and bronchiectasis have chronic sputum production, they usually do not require antibiotic therapy. However, when symptoms of cough, sputum production, and dyspnea become so severe that they interfere with the patient's daily performance, "suppressive" antibiotic therapy is helpful. The first-line antibiotics (see above) are used on a once-daily basis for 10 to 14 days and may be rotated every 2 to 4 weeks. Symptomatic superinfection with gram-negative organisms requires therapy with either third-generation cephalosporins or the quinolones.

Community-Acquired Pneumonia

The most serious infectious complication of COPD is pneumonia. In contrast to acute and chronic bronchitis, patients with pneumonia experience worsening symptoms of cough, but with fever, intense dyspnea, and chest discomfort. Posteroanterior and lateral chest radiographs should be done. Because of the anatomical alterations caused by COPD, the chest x-ray may not demonstrate a typical lobar pattern with dense alveolar consolidation. Also, a "Swiss-cheese lung," mimicking a necrotizing pneumonia, may be apparent.

(continued)

Table 5 Outpatient Pneumonia with Comorbidity

60 Years of Age or Older[1,2]

Organisms:
S. pneumoniae
Respiratory viruses
H. influenzae
Aerobic gram-negative baccilli
S. aureus
Miscellaneous; *E. Pneumoniae, Mycoplasma, Moraxella catarrhalis, Legionella sp., M. tuberculosis,* endemic fungi

Therapy:
Second-generation cephalosporin
OR
Trimethoprim-sulfamethoxazole
OR
Beta-lactam/beta-lactamase inhibitor ±
Erythromycin or other macrolide[3]

[1] Excludes patients at risk for HIV.
[2] In roughly one-third to one-half of the cases no etiology was identified.
[3] If infection with Legionella sp. is a concern.

Establishing the etiology of pneumonia in patients with COPD is often difficult. Routine examination of sputum with gram stain and culture is not always helpful. Some patients are unable to produce adequate sputum samples. In others, the organisms identified may not represent the pathogen. The most common etiological agents along with suggested therapies are listed in Table 5. Although pneumococcal pneumonia remains common, gram-negative organisms (some of which produce beta-lactamase) may be the major pathogens in patients who have recently been hospitalized, who reside in nursing homes, or who have been on previous antibiotic therapy. Pneumococcal vaccine is recommended.

Since the severity of illness is greater in COPD patients with pneumonia, broad-spectrum antibiotics (including second- and third-generation antibiotics, newer macrolide antibiotics, and quinolones) should be used. Many patients require hospitalization because of acute respiratory failure (See Section H.4) and should receive the above antibiotics intravenously. In critical patients, aminoglycosides or third-generation cephalosporins, vancomycin, and erythromycin should be administered until a specific etiology is identified.

The "atypical" pneumonias are emerging as important causes of disease in patients with COPD. These include *Legionella, Chlamydia pneumoniae, Moraxella catarrhalis,* and *Mycoplasma pneumoniae*. If tolerated, erythromycin remains the drug of choice. Newer macrolides such as clarithromycin and azithromycin are excellent but more expensive. For patients allergic to macrolides, quinolones, or doxycycline should be used.

Viral infections may cause atypical pneumonia and acute exacerbations of COPD. The resolution of viral pneumonia can be complicated by residual bronchiolitis and bronchiectasis and by increased airflow obstruction. Influenza can be a fatal illness, and all patients with COPD should be given annual influenza vaccinations. While cytomegalovirus and herpes simplex may occur, this usually only happens in patients who are immunosuppressed with large doses of corticosteroids.

Mycobacterial Disease

There has been a dramatic worldwide increase in the incidence of tuberculosis over the past decade. Patients with underlying COPD seem to be more susceptible to atypical mycobacterial disease, and one should always consider the diagnosis of tuberculosis in patents whose chest x-rays show cavitary apical disease. In addition, a nonresolving or slowly progressing infiltrate can be caused by *Mycobacterium tuberculosis*. Once suspicious of mycobacterial disease, the physician should proceed with the following diagnostic studies:

1. Sputum examination for acid fast bacilli, (AFB), smear and cultures.
2. Placement of intermediate strength purified protein derivative, (PPD).
3. Possible bronchoscopy for cultural and histological examinations of bronchial washing, brushing, and biopsy.

Fungal Infections

Fungi remain an important consideration in the differential diagnosis of certain infiltrates in patients with COPD. Depending on geography, specific fungal pathogens must be considered. In the Ohio and Mississippi River Valleys, *histoplasmosis* is endemic and may cause acute or chronic disease. In the southwestern United States (California and Arizona), *coccidioido-mycosis* is endemic and can be epidemic following a dust storm. Patients may present with acute respiratory illness with or without pulmonary infiltrates.

Aspergillus is a pathogen that can be extremely dangerous in patients with COPD. Individuals on long-term corticosteroid therapy who have been colonized with *Aspergillus* are at higher risk for the "semi-invasive" form of infection. Treatment for this difficult disease requires subspecialty consultation and prolonged intravenous therapy. Rarely, patients with COPD may have an element of allergic broncho-pulmonary aspergillosis, but this is usually limited to patients with asthma.

Because of the difficulty in determining the significance of sputum cultures positive for fungi (i.e., infection versus colonization), consultation is usually recommended before initiating specific antifungal therapy. ■

References

Adams WG, Berk SL. *Moraxella catarrhalis:* An emerging pathogen. J Respir Dis 1993;14:1352-1360. This article emphasizes that *M. catarrhalis,* formerly known as *Neisseria catarrhalis*, is an important pulmonary pathogen in some patients with COPD.

Fein AM, Feinsilver SH, Niederman MS. Nonresolving and slowly resolving pneumonia. Clin Chest Med 1993;14:555-569. This review emphasizes the cause of the slow resolution of pneumonic infiltrations. COPD is one cause of slowly resolving pneumonia.

Mandell GH, Bennett JG, Dolan R. *Principles and Practices of Infectious Disease.* Churchill-Livingstone: New York, 1995 (4th edition). This full-length text is a general reference on the treatment of infectious disease, including those involving the lungs.

Niederman MS, Campbell GD, Fein AM, et al. Guidelines for the initial management of adults with community-acquired pneumonia: Diagnosis, assessment of severity, and initial antimicrobial therapy. Am Rev Respir Dis 1993;148:1418-1426. A current set of guidelines for the management of acquired pneumonias, including those encountered in patients with COPD.

Treatment Complications

H.2 Surgical Procedures

The decision regarding surgery in the COPD patient must weigh the necessity of the proposed procedure against the potential risk to the patient. Any patient with moderate to severe COPD is at increased risk for postoperative complications, particularly respiratory complications. Patients having thoracic or abdominal surgery are at highest risk, while the risk associated with operations on the extremities is relatively low. With appropriate preparation and good anesthetic technique, most operations can be completed successfully and the risk of postoperative complications reduced.

If a given surgery does not involve lung resection and is clearly lifesaving, there is no absolute contraindication to surgery based on pulmonary function. In fact, no level of pulmonary function is an absolute contra-indication to elective nonthoracic surgery that may result in a marked improvement in quality of life. However, a clearly elective procedure with minor implications for improving nonpulmonary function may not be justified in a patient with very severe airflow obstruction.

Preoperative Assessment

A preoperative assessment of the respiratory system in the patient with COPD should include spirometry and arterial blood gas measurements to quantitate the degree of abnormality and to document reversibility. Patients with very severe disease (FEV_1 of approximately 1 liter or less) and those being considered for thoracic surgery, especially if resection of the lung is involved, require more extensive pulmonary function testing. Referral to a pulmonary specialist for this purpose is recommended. Evaluation for lung resection should generally follow the algorithm shown in Figure 6.

Preoperative Management

Long-range preparation (beginning several weeks before the operation) should include smoking cessation, if this has not already been achieved. Bronchodilator therapy should be optimized as described in Section G. This should include a short trial of oral prednisone in

Figure 6 Evaluation for Lung Resection

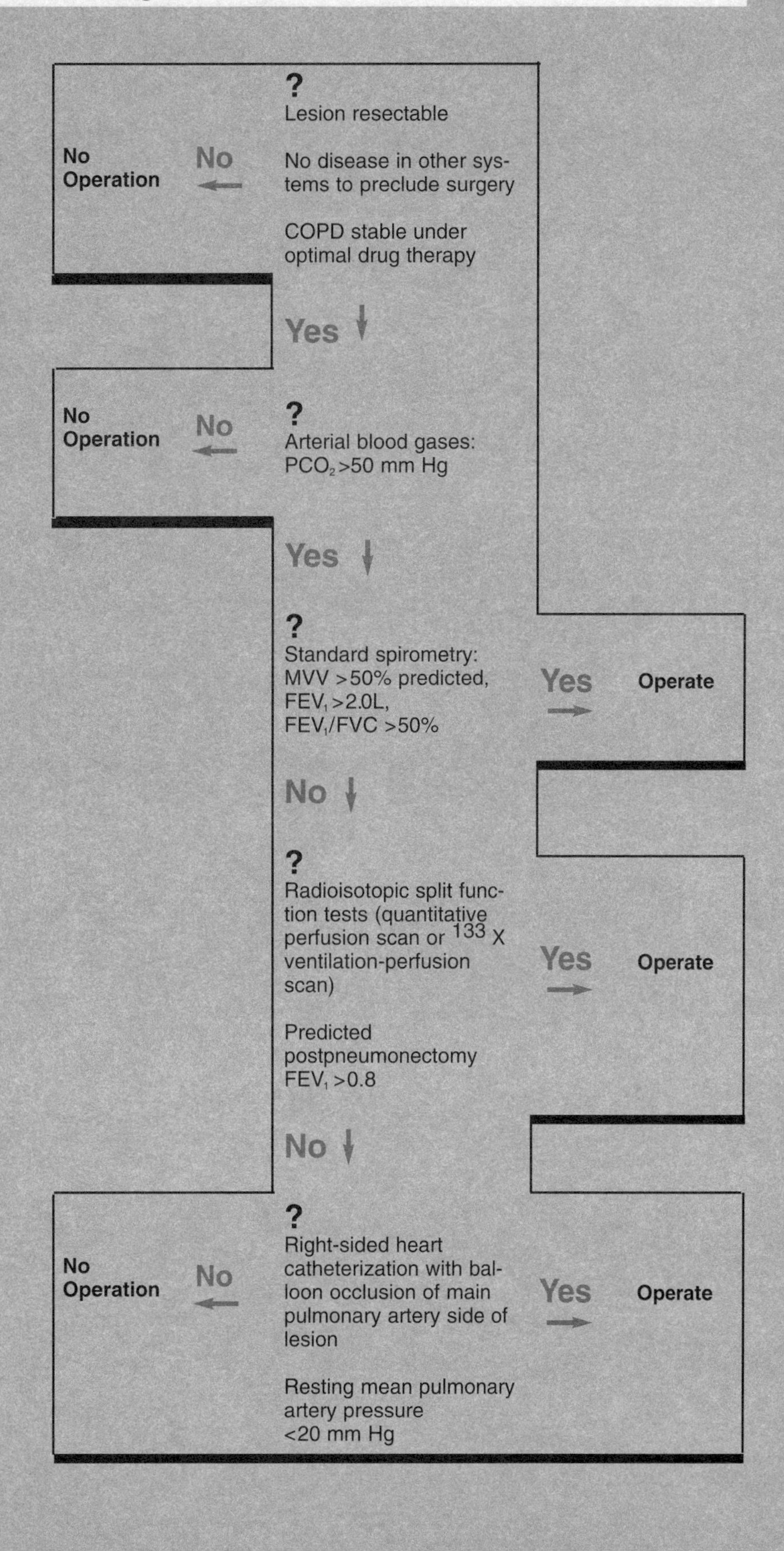

patients with severe disease (FEV_1 <50% of predicted). Secretion clearance should also be optimized by ordering a trial of chest physiotherapy and teaching the patient the proper technique for coughing after the inhalation of bronchodilators. Any measures that might be required postoperatively, including the use of incentive spirometry, should be introduced preoperatively.

Perioperative Management

The anesthesiologist should be alerted that the patient is a high-risk patient and should plan the anesthesia accordingly. Usually the procedure should be scheduled later in the day to allow the patient sufficient time to clear the night's accumulated secretions before being given preoperative medications. Intravenous corticosteroids are indicated perioperatively if the patient has been receiving corticosteroids preoperatively; 50 to 100 mg of prednisolone or an equivalent delivered intravenously is a common loading dose prior to surgery.

Postoperative Management

Attention to postoperative analgesia is extremely important to allow effective coughing. Epidural analgesia and patient-controlled analgesia are particularly useful techniques. Extubation of the patient as soon as possible is recommended to restore the patient's ability to cough. Frequent deep breathing to counteract atelectasis and coughing to clear secretions should be encouraged.

Incentive spirometry is a convenient technique to encourage deep breathing. Early ambulation and mobilization following surgery are especially helpful to patients whose compromised respiratory function predisposes them to pulmonary complications. If immobilization is unavoidable, efforts should be made to turn the patient often and the use of a rotating bed should be considered.

Recently, resection of the lung to improve the functioning of the remaining lung (possibly by eliminating excessive volume and partially restoring elastic recoil aimed at a more effective position of the diaphragm) has been proposed to improve dyspnea in patients with severe COPD. Further experience with this procedure is warranted before it can be recommended for routine use and particularly before patients can be appropriately selected.

Lung Volume Reduction Surgery, (LVRS)

The history of lung volume reduction surgery, (LVRS), is interesting. In the late 1950's, an operation to improve pulmonary function by resecting areas of severest damage from emphysema, was introduced by Brantigan. Although clinical benefit occurred in some patients, operative and postoperative complications caused surgeons to abandon this somewhat heroic operation in that era. Joel Cooper, who was one of the main pioneers in lung transplantation, reopened the issue of clinical and physiological improvements in the modern era and showed substantial benefits in selected patients. Since most of the candidates for LVRS were elderly Medicare patients, the Health Care Finance Administration in conjunction with the National Heart, Lung, and Blood Institute have mandated a randomized controlled clinical trial comparing pulmonary rehabilitation with initial pulmonary rehabilitation following by LVRS. The purpose of this study is to identify the candidates most likely to benefit physiologically, to determine whether or not the surgery has an acceptable perioperative morbidity and mortality, and if survival is altered by this technique. This study is know as the National Emphysema Therapy Trial, (NETT). It will be perhaps five to ten years before the results of the NETT are completed.

Lung Transplantation

Lung transplantation is clearly established as beneficial for advanced stages of COPD. The limitation of organ availability, makes this dramatic surgery available to only a small minority of patients with advanced COPD, mostly of the emphysema type. ■

References

Bartlett RH. Respiratory therapy to prevent pulmonary complications of surgery. Respir Care 1984;29:667-679. This article is one of several published in two issues of Respiratory Care (May and June, 1984) from a symposium that dealt with perioperative respiratory care.

Boysen PG. Perioperative management of the thoracotomy patient. Clin Chest Med 1993;14:321-333. This article is included in a highly recommended issue of Clinics in Chest Medicine dedicated to perioperative care. This particular article focuses on preoperative and intraoperative management aimed at improving pulmonary function during the postoperative period.

Brantigan OC, Kress M, Mueller E. The surgical approach to pulmonary emphysema. Dis Chest 1961;39:485-499. The description of Brantigan's operative procedure designed to improve the elastic recoil in the lungs of patients with advanced emphysema.

Cooper JD, Patterson GA, Sundaresan RS, et al. Results of 150 consecutive bilateral lung volume reduction procedures in patients with severe emphysema. J Thorac Cardiovasc Surg 1996;112:1319-1333. Limited results of the lung volume reduction surgery series from the St. Louis group.

Cooper JD, Trulock EP, Triantafillou AN, et al. Bilateral pneumectomy (volume reduction) for chronic obstructive pulmonary disease. J Thorac Cardiovasc Surg 1995;109:106-119. The first report from the St. Louis group on the modern approach to lung volume reduction surgery.

Davis RD, Jr., Trulock EP, Manley J, et al. Differences in early results after single-lung transplantation. Ann

Thorac Surg 1994;58:1327-1334. Report of 43 COPD patients of 83 single lung transplantations for all causes in the St. Louis series.

Hudson LD, Pierson DJ, Pavlin EG. Evaluation and management of the patient with lung disease who requires surgery. in Kelley W (ed). *Textbook of Internal Medicine, Second Edition.* Philadelphia: JB Lippincott Company, 1992, pp 1865-1870. This chapter is a succinct review of how to evaluate (in order to establish their increased risk for postoperative complications) and subsequently manage the patient with lung disease who requires surgery.

Luce JM. Clinical risk factors for postoperative pulmonary complications. Respir Care 1984;29:484-495. A review of the variables that predispose a patient to an increased risk of developing postoperative pulmonary complications.

Marshall MC, Olsen GN. The physiologic evaluation of the lung resection candidate. Clin Chest Med 1993;14:305-320. A thorough review of the evaluation procedures and techniques designed to predict postoperative morbidity and mortality.

Yeager MP, Glass DD, Neff RK, et al. Epidural anesthesia and analgesia in high risk surgical patients. Anesthesiology 1987;66:729-736. A report of a randomized controlled clinical trial that demonstrated beneficial effects of epidural anesthesia and postoperative analgesia (EAA), on postoperative morbidity in a group of high-risk surgical patients.

Zibrak JD, O'Donnell CR. Indications for preoperative pulmonary function testing. Clin Chest Med 1993; 14:227-236. This article discusses the controversies surrounding the use of preoperative pulmonary function testing to identify high-risk surgical candidates.

Treatment Complications

H.3 Sleep Disorders

Nocturnal oxygen desaturation in COPD patients is fairly common and often unrecognized. It is not usually caused by sleep apnea. Instead, sleep-related hypoxemia has been attributed to ventilation-perfusion abnormalities and transient hypoventilation during rapid eye movement, (REM), sleep. Nonobese patients with COPD who have daytime normoxemia and transient nocturnal hypoxemia during sleep rarely develop coexisting upper airway obstruction or "obstructive sleep apnea." But in some obese individuals with COPD an "overlap syndrome" occurs, adding an obstructive component to the typical mechanisms of transient hypoxemia.

Sleep-related hypoxemia is suggested by the presence of an expanded red cell mass as reflected by an increased hematocrit, along with a patient's reports of morning headaches and daytime somnolence. Often, the patient's spouse is aware of intense snoring and even chooses to sleep in a separate room because of it. The spouse may also notice pauses in breathing followed by loud bursts of snoring when breathing resumes. These reports strongly suggest obstructive sleep apnea.

Diagnosis

Sleep-related hypoxemia and its mechanisms can be diagnosed via overnight home monitoring with a pulse oximeter. The pulse oximeter should be equipped with a memory system and a device to observe whether chest motion ceases during episodes of hypoxemia. Such pauses indicate that a coexisting obstructive component is present. Home sleep studies must be ordered and interpreted by a qualified specialist. Formal polysomnography can provide additional information about the mechanisms associated with nocturnal hypoxemia, but such studies are expensive and must be conducted in a sleep lab, an unusual sleeping environment.

Treatment

Whether or not nocturnal hypoxemia should be treated with oxygen supplementation has been the subject of numerous studies. Two controlled clinical trials in patients with daytime normoxemia (PaO_2 >60 mm Hg) showed a better survival rate in those who did not experience nocturnal desaturation compared with those who did. These studies also showed a trend toward increased survival in oxygen-treated desaturators, compared with desaturators who breathed room air. In fact, one double-blind trial of nocturnal oxygen supplementation for sleep desaturation in patients with daytime normoxemia showed an approximate 4 mm Hg reduction in pulmonary arterial pressures in those treated with oxygen. In contrast, patients who breathed only room air had an increase in their mean pulmonary arterial pressure of approximately 4 mm Hg.

At the present time, experts plan to conduct additional controlled clinical trials to determine whether or not mortality in COPD can be reduced when nocturnal desaturation is treated with oxygen. The outcomes of these studies will answer remaining questions about prescribing nocturnal oxygen.

In light of our current knowledge in this area, what should primary care physicians do if nocturnal desaturation is suspected? If home monitoring with a pulse oximeter identifies nocturnal hypoxemia ($SaO_2 < 88\%$), and if symptoms of headache, fatigue, and poor exercise tolerance are present, it would be wise for the physician to prescribe home oxygen at a liter-flow rate sufficient to correct the hypoxemia. The oxygen "dose" can be determined by studying pulse oximeter readouts taken over several nights while the patient breathes supplemental oxygen. The physician should also ask the patient to report any symptom improvements. In the case of overlap syndrome, providing continuous positive airway pressure, (CPAP), via a well-fitting nasal mask can also be beneficial.

Caution should be used in prescribing sedative agents for insomnia in COPD patients, and patients should be warned against excessive alcohol consumption. Some of these agents may cause disordered sleep patterns and, in extreme cases, might depress respiration, thus augmenting nocturnal hypoventilation. ■

References

Block AJ, Boysen PG, Wynne JW. The origins of cor pulmonale: A hypothesis. Chest 1979;75:109-110. This editorial suggests that nocturnal hypoxemia and resultant hypoxemic pulmonary vasoconstriction indicate early stages of pulmonary hypertension in COPD.

Catterall JR, Douglas NJ, Calverley PMA, et al. Transient hypoxemia during sleep in chronic obstructive pulmonary disease is not a sleep apnea syndrome. Am Rev Respir Dis 1983;128:24-29. This articles gives evidence that nocturnal hypoxemia is usually caused by factors other than sleep apnea.

Flenley DC. Sleep in chronic lung disease. Clin Chest Med 1986;6:652-658. An overlap syndrome of concurrent nocturnal hypoxemia in COPD and sleep apnea is discussed here.

Fletcher EC, Donner CF, Midgren B, et al. Survival in COPD patients with a daytime PaO_2 >60 Torr with and without nocturnal oxyhemoglobin desaturation (NOD). Chest 1992;101:649-655. This study shows the adverse prognosis of patients with isolated nocturnal oxygen desaturation compared with patients who do not have nocturnal oxygen desaturation.

Fletcher EC, Luckett RA, Goodnight-White S, et al. A double-blind trial of nocturnal supplemental oxygen for sleep desaturation in patients with chronic obstructive pulmonary disease and a daytime PaO_2 above 60 Torr. Am Rev Respir Dis 1992;145:1070-1076. A favorable effect of nocturnal oxygen administration on survival in nocturnal desaturations is suggested by this study.

Treatment Complications

H.4 Acute Respiratory Failure

Acute respiratory failure, (ARF), is a severe complication in the patient with COPD. ARF is broadly defined as an acute worsening of blood gases to a degree that represents a threat to life. The exact definition may vary but usually consists of a significant and sudden change from the baseline arterial blood gas values to a PCO_2 >50 mm Hg with a pH of <7.30 and/or a PO_2 <50 mm Hg.

Diagnosis

ARF presents as a deterioration in clinical status, usually the onset or worsening of respiratory symptoms such as cough and dyspnea. However, central nervous system symptoms, including irritability or drowsiness, may be the most prominent. Presenting symptoms may also reflect the acute condition which precipitates the ARF. For example, complications caused by a respiratory infection can include an exacerbation of bronchitis or pneumonia. A variety of other conditions, including congestive heart failure or any systemic condition which increases metabolic demands, may contribute. Once the diagnosis is suspected, it should be confirmed by obtaining arterial blood gases analyses.

Prognosis

The prognosis of ARF in the COPD patient is better than commonly believed. Approximately 90% of patients survive the acute episode. Prognosis following ARF depends on the underlying lung function and is no different for a patient who has had ARF compared to one who has not, provided that their FEV_1 values are the same.

Treatment

Patients with ARF generally require hospitalization, but less severe exacerbations can be treated in the outpatient setting according to the steps described in Section G. The treatment of ARF in any patient has four objectives: 1) The correction of physiologic abnormalities–with the correction of hypoxemia using supplemental oxygen being especially important; 2) aggressive treatment of airflow obstruction, including bronchodilator therapy, administration of

Table 6 Management of Acute Respiratory Failure with COPD

1. Correct Physiologic Abnormalities

A. Correct life-threatening hypoxemia:

1. Usually requires only small increase in FIO_2 (1 to 2 L/min by nasal prongs).
2. Infiltrate or pulmonary edema suggests the presence of a shunt, and a higher FIO_2 may be required.
3. Usually the therapeutic goal is a PaO_2 of 55 to 65 mm Hg (associated with nearly complete oxygen saturation of hemoglobin).
4. Observe for signs of CO_2 retention and check arterial blood gases after increments in FIO_2.

B. Correct life-threatening respiratory acidosis:

1. Usually is less urgent than correcting hypoxemia.
2. Usually is accomplished with therapy to improve airflow and to remove secretions.
3. Decision to use mechanical ventilation depends more on clinical status (especially mental status) than level of pH or PCO_2.
4. Bicarbonate therapy is rarely indicated.

2. Treat Airflow Obstruction

A. Treatment aimed at bronchodilation and control of inflammation:

1. First-line: Use inhaled ipratropium and beta-agonist; intravenous corticosteroids.
2. Second-line: Use theophylline.

B. Treatment aimed at improving secretion removal:

Use hydration, chest percussion, inhaled heated moisture as indicated.

3. Treat Precipitating Events As Indicated (e.g., Acute Purulent Bronchitis, Pneumonia, Congestive Heart Failure)

4. Prevent Complications

A. Cardiac dysrhythmias: maintain oxygenation and normalize electrolyte values; monitor level of theophylline, if used.

B. Pulmonary thromboembolism: use subcutaneous heparin for prophylaxis, if not contraindicated.

C. Treat gastrointestinal complications. Prophylaxis of gastrointestinal bleeding: sucralfate, Nasogastric suctioning, if aerophagia is a problem.

D. Nosocomial infection: use sucralfate for prophylaxis of gastrointestinal bleeding.

Treatment
(continued)

corticosteroids, and the removal of airway secretions; 3) treatment for the factor precipitating ARF; and 4) the prevention of complications. In addition to these, mechanical ventilation may be required in a minority of patients. Important points regarding these aspects of management are summarized in Table 6.

Correcting life-threatening hypoxemia is particularly important. The goal of oxygen therapy is to achieve an arterial oxygen saturation above 90%, which generally means an arterial PO_2 of approximately 60 mm Hg. Usually a small amount of supplemental oxygen (1 to 2 liters per minute via nasal prongs) will suffice to provide this level of oxygenation. Higher amounts of supplemental oxygen may be necessary if the patient has a significant right-to-left shunt, which may be associated with pneumonia or congestive heart failure. Although progressive respiratory acidosis can complicate oxygen administration in ARF, the incidence of this complication has been overemphasized. More importantly, if O_2 therapy is prudently administered and monitored by repeated measurements of arterial blood, the therapeutic goal can be achieved without a significant CO_2 increase in nearly all patients.

Treating a potentially reversible component of airflow obstruction is one of the most important aspects of therapy. Even when a patient has not responded to bronchodilation during their stable state, he or she may display a reversible obstructive component during ARF. Therefore, inhaled bronchodilators should be given aggressively and should include inhaled ipratropium bromide and an inhaled beta-agonist. Corticosteroids should be given, initially intravenously as methylprednisolone sodium succinate, at least 125 mg/day in divided doses. Oral prednisone may be given later (60 mg/day with a gradual taper from that dose) once it is assured that the patient is able to eat and does not have an ileus. Intravenous aminophylline should be given in an average maintenance dose of 0.6 mg/kg/hr in patients already receiving oral theophylline. If the patient has not significantly improved within 12 to 24 hours with inhaled bronchodilators and intravenous corticosteroids and has not been receiving oral theophylline, intravenous theophylline should be added in a loading dose of 3 to 5 mg/kg to be followed by the above-described maintenance dose.

Also, since most patients with acute respiratory failure have problems with retained secretions, these should be addressed therapeutically. Treatment for retained secretions consists primarily of adequate hydration (not overhydration) and encouraging the patient to cough (sitting upright in a position that enhances the ability to cough) following a dose of inhaled bronchodilators.

Specific treatment for any recognized precipitating factors should be given. Broad-spectrum antibiotics are required when there is even the slightest suspicion of bacterial bronchitis or if pneumonia is diagnosed, as discussed in Section H.1.

Mechanical ventilation may be needed in a minority (approximately 10%) of COPD patients with ARF. The decision to use mechanical ventilation is based primarily on clinical grounds rather than any particular level of blood gas abnormalities. Worsening mental status with an onset of lethargy, confusion, and somnolence–despite aggressive administration of the above therapies–is the primary indication. If one is not experienced in supervising mechanical ventilation, consultation with a pulmonary specialist is warranted. Some aspects of mechanical ventilation of particular importance in the COPD patient are outlined in Table 7. Alternatives to intubation and mechanical ventilation (e.g., noninvasive ventilation using a face mask) are currently being explored and should be considered only if expertise with these techniques is locally available (See below).

The possibility of endotracheal intubation and mechanical ventilation should be discussed with each patient with severe COPD and his or her family while

Treatment *(continued)*

stable (as an outpatient) to establish directives regarding the patient's wishes. If there is an acute precipitating cause which is potentially reversible, then prognosis with mechanical ventilation is favorable. Frequently, however, no readily reversible component can be identified, but even then patients may respond favorably. Therefore, it is recommended that you discuss whether or not to withdraw support if the patient does not improve after many days of aggressive treatment. This option allows the chance for successful treatment for ARF, but also allows patients to avoid a situation that many fear: that they will require prolonged mechanical ventilation that may not be compatible with an acceptable quality of life. If the decision is made to withdraw mechanical ventilatory support, the goal of treatment becomes patient comfort. Narcotics should be given as needed.

Noninvasive Mechanical Ventilation

In recent years, the technique of noninvasive mechanical ventilation has begun to replace more invasive mechanical ventilation with intubation. Thus, with tight-fitting, comfortable face masks, and practical, safe, home mechanical ventilators, noninvasive positive pressure breathing is commonly used both in hospitals and within the home, in the short-term to deal with exacerbations of COPD. Some patients can achieve rest and restoration of respiratory muscle function during short periods of nocturnal mechanical ventilation during either positive pressure breathing or non-invasively, without a mask, with negative pressure mechanical ventilation using body wrap or cuirass-type ventilators. It is stressed that noninvasive mechanical ventilation only assists the patient's efforts in breathing, and cannot be used to take over the complete ventilatory support of patients. Nonetheless, non-invasive mechanical ventilation will replace intubation with mechanical ventilation in an increasing number of patients in the future, as techniques improve. ■

Table 7 Management of Acute Respiratory Failure

Management of Acute Respiratory Failure in Selected Patients Requiring Mechanical Ventilation

Institute Mechanical Ventilation If Mental Status Deteriorates
A. Prevent barotrauma and impaired cardiac output because of intrinsic PEEP on mechanical ventilation.
1. Use modest tidal volume (7 to 8 mL/kg).
2. Minimize VE, peak, and mean airway pressures.
B. If intrinsic PEEP develops, attempt to:
1. Decrease respiratory rate.
2. Increase inspiratory flow rate (approximately 5 to 6 x VE).
3. Decrease tidal volume.
4. Try pressure support.

PEEP=Positive end expiratory pressure

References

Albert RK, Martin TR, Lewis SW. Controlled clinical trial of methylprednisolone in patients with chronic bronchitis and acute respiratory insufficiency. Ann Int Med 1980; 92:753-758. This well-controlled clinical trial showed an objective improvement in FEV_1 with corticosteroid use compared with placebo. The differences were small but statistically significant.

American Thoracic Society. Withholding and withdrawing life sustaining therapy. Am Rev Respir Dis 1989;140 (Part 2):S1-S107. This is a detailed report of a NIH-sponsored workshop, "Withholding and Withdrawing Mechanical Ventilation."

Chevrolet JC, Jolliet P, Abajo B, et al. Nasal positive pressure ventilation in patients with acute respiratory failure. Difficult and time-consuming procedure for nurses. Chest 1991; 100:775-782. This report on the use of a noninvasive method of mechanical ventilation found it time consuming and not effective in interstitial fibrosis.

Curtis JR, Hudson LD. Emergent assessment and management of acute respiratory failure in COPD. Clin Chest Med 1994;15:481-500. This is a state-of-the-art review of contemporary strategies for the management of acute respiratory failure.

Derenne J, Fleury B, Pariente R. Acute respiratory failure of chronic obstructive pulmonary disease. Am Rev Respir Dis 1988; 138:1006-1033. This is a complete review of the pathophysiology and treatment of acute respiratory failure in COPD.

Karpel JP. Bronchodilator responses to anticholinergic and beta-adrenergic agents in acute and stable COPD. Chest 1991; 99:871-876. This study showed that ipratropium and metaproterenol were equally effective in the doses used.

Treatment Complications

H.5 Cor Pulmonale

Cor pulmonale literally means "the heart of the lungs." Its formal pathological definition is "right ventricular enlargement, hypertrophy, or dilation, secondary to lung disease." To understand cor pulmonale, one must appreciate the physiology of the normal pulmonary circulatory system and its response to disease.

Pathophysiology

As described elsewhere in this monograph, COPD is, in most patients, a mixture of two or three related pulmonary diseases. These include asthmatic bronchitis and chronic bronchitis, which involve inflammation of the airways, bronchi, and bronchioles; and pulmonary emphysema, which affects the lung parenchyma through destruction of alveolar walls and their associated capillary circulatory framework.

In emphysema, the capillary bed is progressively and irreversibly destroyed, which eventually raises pulmonary vascular resistance and pulmonary artery pressure. Persistent and worsening pulmonary hypertension, in turn, finally results in cor pulmonale. Cor pulmonale usually appears only in the very advanced stages of emphysema.

In both chronic bronchitis and asthmatic bronchitis, however, pulmonary hypertension may occur much earlier in the course of disease than in emphysema. When hypoxemia, hypercarbia, and acidosis develop in chronic bronchitis, they cause pulmonary artery vasoconstriction, which increases pulmonary vascular resistance and, again, results in pulmonary hypertension that leads to irreversible vascular changes. Chronic severe hypoxemia is invariably present, often associated with secondary erythrocytosis.

If untreated, the increased pulmonary artery pressure will eventually "overload" the right ventricle. The normal heart's first response is to expand the size of the right ventricular muscle. This hypertrophy can compensate for mild pressure overloads for months or even years. Eventually, however, the heart dilates, and symptoms of right-sided heart failure or decompensated cor pulmonale (elevated neck veins, congested liver, and peripheral edema) appear.

At this stage, pulmonary artery pressures are usually elevated above 25/15 mm Hg, and they may reach as high as 60/30 mm Hg, although this is rare. (Normal pulmonary artery pressure in a young person at rest averages 15/8 mm Hg; the upper limit of normal is 25/15 mm Hg.) The right ventricle fails and further pulmonary artery pressure elevation to systemic levels does not occur as it does in primary pulmonary hypertension. The reason for a relatively modest increase in pulmonary hypertension in COPD and the heart's failure to increase its right ventricular mass to deal with rising pulmonary vascular resistance is not known.

Clinical Diagnosis

If a patient presents with peripheral edema, elevation of the neck veins, and a congested liver, one can make a clinical diagnosis of right-sided heart failure. If such a patient has a significant degree of COPD and an elevated hematocrit with hypoxemia as outlined above, the diagnosis of cor pulmonale as a complication of COPD can be made with a high degree of confidence without further expensive tests other than a standard electrocardiogram. More extensive and expensive tests such as echocardiography or right ventricular catheterization should be done only if the patient does not respond to standard therapy as outlined below and/or if there is clinical evidence of additional left-sided heart disease.

Standard Therapy

As discussed throughout this monograph, the basic treatment for all complications of COPD, including cor pulmonale, is to treat the underlying airflow obstruction to improve the patient's oxygenation. Patients with mild heart failure can be managed by restricting their salt intake to 2 g per day and prescribing a good 24-hour diuretic such as hydrochlorothiazide (25 to 50 mg once a day), bumetanide (1 to 2 mg once a day), or furosemide (20 to 40 mg given twice daily). Many clinicians mistakenly prescribe furosemide once in the morning only, which causes patients to excrete salt early in the day but then retain it again after the evening meal.

Oxygen Therapy

If edema cannot be controlled by salt restriction and diuretics, and/or if the patient presents with severe edema and obvious decompensated cor pulmonale, the most essential treatment is supplemental oxygen. Oxygen must be given at whatever flow rate (dosage) and with whatever delivery system required to achieve arterial oxygen saturations in the 90% to 95% range, 24 hours per day.

It is a good practice for the clinician to check follow-up hematocrit or hemoglobin levels at 4 to 8 week intervals. If the patient is being adequately oxygenated, secondary erythrocytosis will resolve within 4 to 8 weeks in almost all patients. Persistent erythrocytosis indicates that the patient is either not using his or her oxygen as much as required, or that desaturation is present during sleep despite the fact that supplementary oxygen is being breathed. In these situations, a sleep study (Discussed in Section H.3) should be performed to see if additional therapy for obstructive sleep disorder is needed and if therapy such as CPAP is required.

(continued)

Digitalis

Time and experience have shown that digitalis is not effective in the treatment of cor pulmonale when it is used without first controlling the patient's underlying hypoxemia and pulmonary hypertension. Once this is done, digitalis is rarely needed. Digitalis is a poor inotropic agent in cor pulmonale, but it still has a role as a chronotropic drug since it helps control ventricular rates in patients with atrial fibrillation or flutter and a fast ventricular response. When left-sided heart failure accompanies right-sided heart failure (see below), digitalis is helpful as an inotropic agent for the left ventricle.

Refractory Cor Pulmonale

If treatment for cor pulmonale as outlined above does not relieve right-sided heart failure, chronic thromboembolic disease or coexisting left-sided heart failure may be present. Diagnosis of these diseases requires additional invasive tests and referral to a specialist is recommended. ■

References

Dunn MI, Galiber DP. When chronic lung disease leads to cor pulmonale. J Respir Dis 1993;14:957-971. This is a review of the pathogenesis and treatment of cor pulmonale associated with COPD.

Galiber DP, Dunn MI. When left heart failure complicates COPD. J Respir Dis 1994;15:475-486. A succinct discussion of the effects of left heart failure on the manifestations and prognosis of COPD.

MacNee W. Pathophysiology of cor pulmonale in chronic obstructive pulmonary disease, part one. Am J Respir Crit Care Med 1994;150:833-852. This is the first part of a detailed state-of-the-art review of the pathogenesis of cor pulmonale.

MacNee W. Pathophysiology of cor pulmonale in chronic obstructive pulmonary disease, part two. Am J Respir Crit Care Med 1994;150:1158-1168. This second part reviews associated left heart failure and the treatment of cor pulmonale. The two articles together contain 519 references!

Neff TA, Petty TL. Long-term continuous oxygen therapy in chronic airway obstruction (CAO). Ann Int Med 1970;72:621-626. This study gives data on the early clinical experiences in Denver using long-term oxygen therapy to treat COPD.

Petty TL (Chairman), Nocturnal Oxygen Therapy Trial Group, (NOTT). Continuous or nocturnal oxygen therapy in hypoxemic chronic obstructive lung disease: A clinical trial. Ann Int Med 1980;93:391-398. This multicenter trial showed better survival with nearly continuous oxygen therapy (average 19.4 hrs/day) compared with nocturnal oxygen therapy (average 11.8 hrs/day).

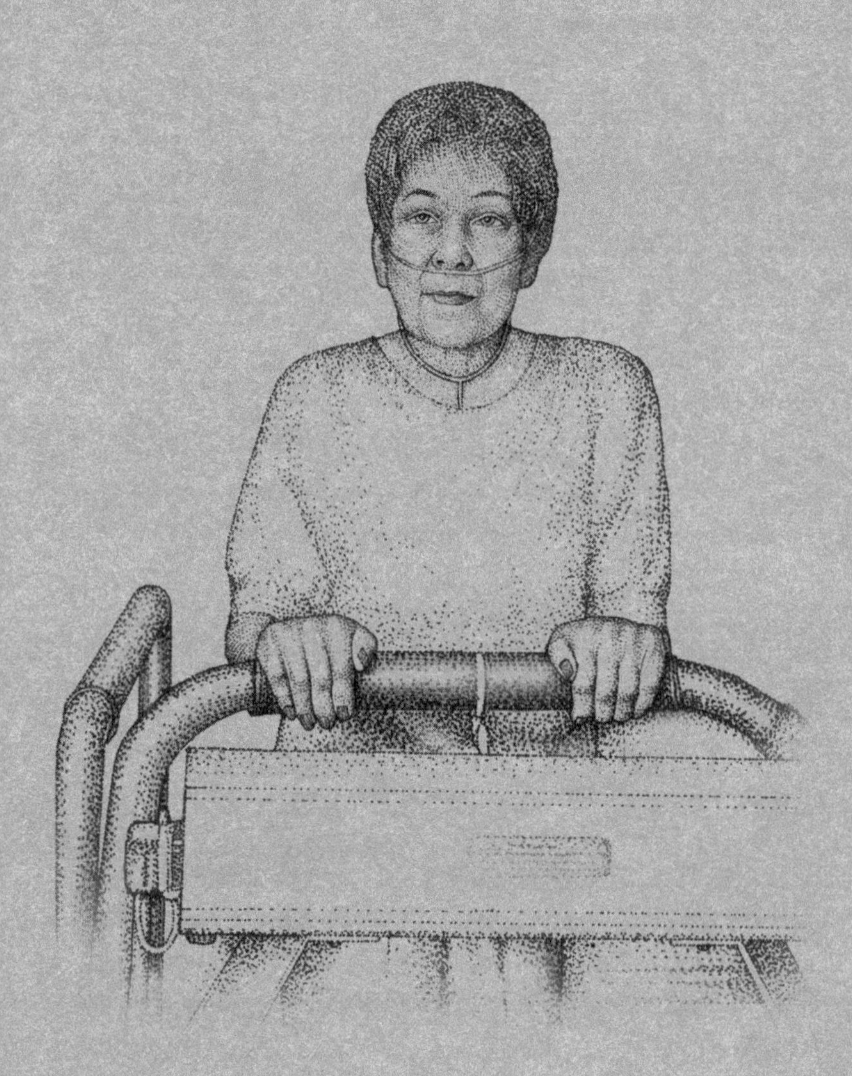

Exercising daily is the key. Walking either outside or on a treadmill, bicycling, swimming, and exercising the upper extremities with barbells, rowing machines, or high reaches are important systemic exercises.

I. Pulmonary Rehabilitation

Pulmonary rehabilitation is a method of systemized, multidisciplinary care that offers significant benefits to many patients with advanced COPD. The roots of pulmonary rehabilitation can be traced to the late 1800's, when tuberculosis was common, scarring the lungs and causing respiratory insufficiency in patients who survived the disease.

The components of pulmonary rehabilitation are:

1. Patient and family education.
2. Smoking cessation.
3. Systemic exercise.
4. Breathing training and exercises.
5. Oxygen therapy in selected patients.
6. Patient support groups.

Pharmacologic agents are also used to treat bronchospasm, improve airflow obstruction, clear mucus, treat infection, and deal with heart failure. But pulmonary rehabilitation consists of much more than ordinary pharmacological management.

Patient and Family Education

Education is the key to rehabilitation in patients with any chronic disorder. COPD patients and their families must understand the basic anatomy and physiology of the lungs and the circulatory system, as well as the concepts of tissue oxygenation, nutrition, exercise physiology, and global health as an alternative to illness. Although patients are stricken with disease, the illness associated with that disease can be minimized through education.

Detailed instructions are provided most efficiently in small group sessions, usually formed at the beginning of a formalized pulmonary rehabilitation program. The interaction of four to six people with similar symptoms and coping problems can provide for a meaningful exchange of information. The preferred method for using a metered-dose inhaler and the roles of other medications in COPD management (See Section G) are taught. Pamphlets and short monographs should also be used to reinforce material presented in these group sessions (See references).

Smoking Cessation

Smoking cessation is critical to the success of pulmonary rehabilitation. Without it, the typical benefits of pulmonary rehabilitation, such as improved symptoms and exercise tolerance, cannot be expected. The relentless progression of airflow obstruction can be dramatically slowed by smoking cessation, even in older individuals who have smoked for 30 to 40 years. It's never too late to stop smoking! (See Section J).

The results of the Lung Health Study re-confirm that smoking cessation has a dramatic effect in slowing the rate of decline of FEV_1, the key indicator of the course and prognosis of COPD. Thus, aggressive attempts at smoking cessation must be made in patients with any degree of airflow obstruction lest progressive disabling disease follows.

Systemic Exercise

Exercise is central to the rehabilitation of respiratory cripples. Even with severe airflow obstruction, i.e., an FEV_1 of less than 1 liter, individuals can learn to walk greater distances without much–or any–distress if they become physically reconditioned. Exercising daily is the key. Walking either outside or on a treadmill, bicycling, swimming, and exercising the upper extremities with barbells, rowing machines, or high reaches are important systemic exercises. Walking out of doors is the most beneficial and pleasant, and is certainly more useful than any form of contrived exercise. But, of course, any exercise is better than none.

Breathing Training and Breathing Exercises

Special breathing techniques, including pursed-lip breathing (Figure 7), also help mitigate dyspnea. Extensive studies have shown that the use of pursed-lip breathing results in a slower, deeper ventilatory pattern that improves oxygenation, probably by improving ventilation-perfusion matching within the lungs. Breathing against a flow or threshold resistor or doing maximum voluntary ventilation maneuvers several times a day has also been shown to strengthen the respiratory muscles. But the increased ventilation required by exercise, especially walking, does the same thing in a more physiological fashion.

Oxygen Therapy

Oxygen therapy is now recognized as a method of care that improves both the length and quality of life in selected patients with advanced COPD. Portable oxygen is available via liquid systems, which are the most popular and practical. Small compressed gas cylinders used with a pulse inspiratory flow device are an alternative. Stationary systems include concentrators and high pressure cylinders (See Table 8).

Portable oxygen can improve exercise capacity and reduce right ventricular strain. Oxygen support during exercise can be integrated into the rehabilitation program for certain patients. Oxygen is generally used when symptomatic patients have a chronic stable PO_2 of 55 mm Hg or less (saturation of 88% or less), but by no means do all patients with this degree of hypoxemia require oxygen. (Otherwise everyone living in Leadville, Colorado, at an elevation of 10,000 feet, would require oxygen!)

Oxygen should be prescribed when patients exhibit dyspnea upon exertion, morning headaches, or evidence of right ventricular strain (as judged by clinical criteria including the presence of electrocardiographic, roentgenographic, and clinical signs suggesting right-sided heart failure or erythrocytosis). In these instances, oxygen tensions as high as 59 mm Hg will qualify for

Figure 7 Pursed-lip Breathing

**Step 1:
Inhale through the nose with the mouth closed.**

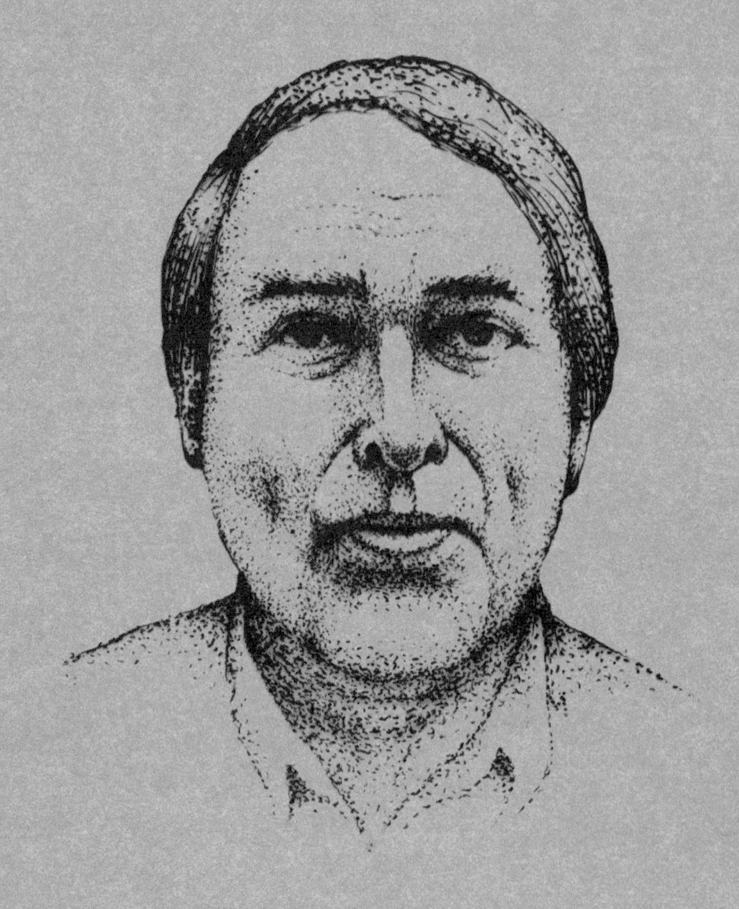

Step 2:
The patient should shape the mouth as though whistling and breathe out slowly, resisting against the force of the air leaving the lungs.

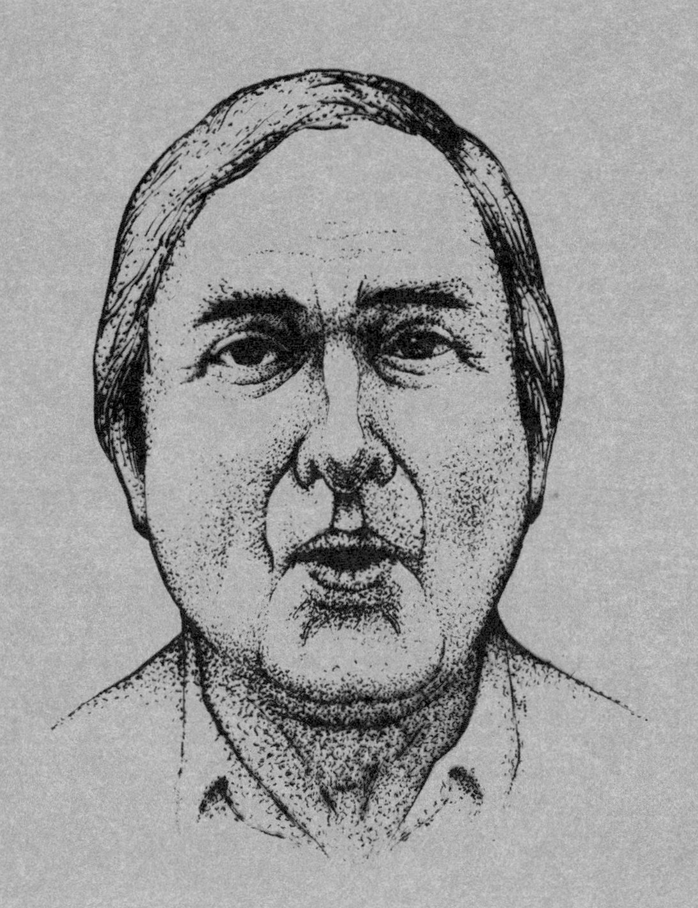

third party reimbursement under Medicare and most insurance plans (See Table 9). Oxygen can sometimes improve exercise tolerance in patients with oxygen tensions of 60 mm Hg or above, probably by providing the additional oxygen required by exercise.

Patient Support Groups

Patient support groups provide an important social outlet for patients and their families. Educational meetings and social outings such as trips on trains, buses, or cruise ships help enhance the quality of life and the happiness of patients with advanced COPD. These groups usually meet on a regular basis, often monthly. At each meeting, a local or outside speaker offers a presentation on a matter of immediate and practical interest; popular discussion topics include human sexuality and coping with sexual dysfunction, diet and nutrition, medications, and medicolegal issues such as advance directives (living wills and durable powers of attorney). A meal, often followed by entertainment, completes the program.

Organization and Structure of a Pulmonary Rehabilitation Program

The great majority of pulmonary rehabilitation programs are provided on an outpatient basis. Referrals usually come from pulmonologists, but today more primary care physicians are referring their patients to 4 to 6 week programs. In all cases, patients remain under the immediate care of their referring physician, who continues to prescribe all medications. Most programs are staffed by 2 to 4 nurses, respiratory therapists, or physical therapists. Daily sessions of 1 to 2 hours are common. Pursed-lip breathing and breathing exercises are demonstrated, then performed by the entire group. Supervised exercise on treadmills and bicycles, with pulse rate and saturation being monitored, is common. Walks around a large room or gymnasium, when available, are also done.

A report of the patient's progress is sent to the referring physician upon completion of the program. "Graduates" are encouraged to continue to participate in the activities of the associated patient support group

Table 8 Home Oxygen Devices Compared

	Portable liquid	Stationary concentrator	Compressed gas
Advantages	Lightweight. Portable canister allows for long-range mobility. Most practical ambulatory system. Valuable for pulmonary rehabilitation. 100% oxygen provided at all flow rates.	Low cost. Convenient for home use. Attractive equipment. Widely available.	Low cost, but may equal the cost of portable liquid when used continuously. Widely available.
Disadvantages	More expensive than concentrator when used alone. Not available in small or rural communities.	Electricity required. May need back-up tank system. Not portable; does not assist in ambulation or in pulmonary rehabilitation. Noisy.	Multiple tanks needed for ambulation, unless transfilling can be done at home. Heavy tanks; not effective in pulmonary rehabilitation. Unsightly equipment.

Table 9 Guidelines for Prescribing Home Oxygen Therapy

The patient has chronic, severe hypoxemia related to:
1. Chronic obstructive pulmonary disease
2. Cystic fibrosis
3. Interstitial lung disease
4. Kyphoscoliosis

Attempts at stabilization with one or more of these agents have failed:
1. Antimicrobial drugs
2. Bronchodilators
3. Corticosteroids
4. Diuretics

One of the following blood gas criteria has been met:
1. Oxygen saturation is <89%.
2. The PO_2 is <56 mm Hg.
3. The PO_2, which is <60 mm Hg, is associated with cor pulmonale, erythrocytosis and a hematrocit >55%, pulmonary hypertension, and/or right ventricular hypertrophy.

as long as they find these sessions valuable. In most cases, graduates continue to participate for years.

Costs for pulmonary rehabilitation vary and may be $2,000 to $4,000 per patient, a gross average. Reimbursement is approved on a regional basis, usually following detailed negotiations with third party payers such as HCFA or HMO's. In most cases, third party payers recognize the tangible cost benefits from pulmonary rehabilitation: fewer hospitalizations, emergency room visits, and clinic visits.

Patients with Early COPD

In the future, pulmonary rehabilitation will probably focus on patients with mild or even asymptomatic disease. It has recently been learned that men with mild COPD have a poor ability to exercise and cannot begin to achieve their maximum oxygen consumption. Poor cardiovascular conditioning results in premature exercise impairment. By contrast, women seem to do better. Further research will determine whether or not exercise training can recondition patients with early COPD. If so, pulmonary rehabilitation techniques should be applied much earlier in the course of COPD than is now the case.

A perspective on the past, present, and future of pulmonary rehabilitation is listed in the References at the end of this Section. ■

References

Anthonisen NR, Connett JE, Kiley JP, et al. Effects of smoking intervention and the use of an inhaled anticholinergic bronchodilator on the rate of decline of FEV_1. JAMA 1994;272:1497-1505. This is the first complete report on the outcomes of the Lung Health Study, which enrolled 5,887 patients aged 35 to 60 (mean 48.5 years) with mild airflow obstruction. Smoking cessation was associated with an improved FEV_1 in younger participants who had the mildest degrees of airflow obstruction. Declines in airflow over five years were much slower in nonsmokers than in continuing smokers.

Petty TL. Pulmonary rehabilitation in perspective: Historical roots, present status and future projections. Thorax 1993;48:855-862. A comprehensive review of the past, present, and future of pulmonary rehabilitation.

Petty TL. Pulmonary rehabilitation: A personal historical perspective. Chapter 1 in Casaburi R, Petty TL (eds). *Principles and Practice of Pulmonary Rehabilitation.* Philadelphia: WB Saunders, 1993. The first chapter of a complete textbook on pulmonary rehabilitation for COPD and other disorders.

Petty TL, Tiep B, Burns M. Essentials of a Pulmonary Rehabilitation Program: A Do It Yourself Program. Part I (1991), Part II (1992), Part III (1993). These are brief pamphlets available from the Pulmonary Education and Research Foundation, PO Box 1133, Lomita CA 90717-5133. (A Spanish version is also available).

J. Prevention

Introduction

Smoking cessation is the most effective treatment for COPD, and the only way to prevent it. The social and economic costs of smoking are enormous. A patient who is successful in stopping smoking will eventually need to be seen less often and hospitalized less frequently, thus reducing a significant portion of these costs.

The Lung Health Study revealed that some patients with early COPD experienced an improvement of pulmonary function after smoking cessation. As already emphasized, this landmark study should encourage every physician to do simple spirometric assessments in all smokers. The rate of decline of pulmonary function was dramatically reduced in patients who stopped smoking in the Lung Health Study. All smokers should quit. Those with decreased pulmonary function are at a particular risk for adverse consequences, including accelerated losses in ventilatory function that result in premature morbidity and mortality from COPD.

The time is ripe for the primary care physician to capitalize on years of public health education about the benefits of smoking cessation. Most persons who smoke know about the economic and health consequences of smoking. The young, however, are especially prone–despite public education efforts–to feel that "it won't happen to me." Some of the many available free smoking cessation resources, appropriate for smokers from all socioeconomic groups, are listed in Tables 10 and 11.

Office Strategy

A physician's office smoking cessation plan need not be complicated, time consuming, or costly. A brief intervention, as short as one or two minutes, can be effective.

The Agency for HealthCare Research and Quality suggests the Five A's approach to smoking cessation intervention. Always **Ask** if the patient smokes, **Advise** smokers to quit, **Assess** the patient's willingness to try to quit, **Assist** the smoker in quitting, and **Arrange** follow-up. Patients expect physicians to advise them to stop, and they will listen. The perception of smokers is that the majority of them have not been told by their physicians to stop smoking!

Any behavioral change progresses through stages. Smokers can be categorized by stage and treated accordingly:

1. Pre-contemplation stage–Smokers at this stage are not seriously considering quitting within six months. Give these smokers pamphlets on the hazards of smoking and the benefits of quitting, which may be obtained from the sources listed in Tables 10 and 11. Tell the patient that you are recording in his or her chart the fact that you have prescribed stopping smoking. Some physicians reinforce this by handing the patient a written prescription for smoking cessation.
2. Contemplation stage–Patients in this stage are seriously considering quitting smoking within six months. Urge them to set a quit date and schedule a visit a month or so prior to that date. Give appropriate smoking information (available from many sources).
3. Preparation stage–This includes those who plan to quit within the next thirty days; they have made a quit attempt lasting 24 hours or longer during the past year. As soon as the patient has set a quit date, evaluate the patient's need for nicotine replacement. Nicotine patches usually double the quit rate and should be considered for nicotine-dependent smokers.

(continued)

The Fagerstrom Nicotine Tolerance Score (Figure 8) is an easy way to evaluate dependence. Patients scoring 6 points or more are highly dependent and will probably need nicotine replacement. A simpler and more practical evaluation method has also been developed; it postulates that the most addicted smokers smoke one to two packs per day and have their first smoke within thirty minutes after arising.

Nicotine patches are easy to explain and cause relatively few problems in addicted patients. Pharmaceutical companies include good information packages along with their products . The American Cancer, Heart, and Lung Associations also provide excellent information (Table 10).

Education about quitting techniques and coping skills improves success. A knowledgeable nurse or assistant can explain techniques and offer reinforcement. This reinforcement can also be very effectively provided during essential follow-up visits at one and three weeks. The best support is understanding guidance, not negative reinforcement. Emphasize that success improves when the patient has a plan to cope with the urge to smoke. If the patient is interested in group sessions, give him or her the number of the local branch of the American Lung Association for information regarding its support groups (Table 10).

Relapse is common in first-time quitters. Approximately 25% succeed, so 75% need to try again. The good news is that success increases with each effort! Encourage the patient to view each unsuccessful quit attempt as a single step in the learning process. Help the patient to see relapse as a trial rather than a failure.

Even those who succeed in quitting tobacco use need continuing support and encouragement from their families and from you and your staff. The primary care physician, is therefore a catalyst for an ongoing process that may last years. *(continued)*

Table 10 Smoking Cessation Information Resources

American Cancer Society	1-800-ACS-2345	www.cancer.org
American Heart Association	1-800-242-1793 1-800-AHA-USA1	www.americanheart.org
American Lung Association	1-800-586-4872 1-800-Lung-USA	www.lungusa.org
Nicotine Anonymous	1-415-750-0328	www.nicotine-anonymous.org
Office on Smoking and Health	1-800-CDC-1311	www.cdc.gov/health/smoking.htm
Surgeon General's Office	1-301-594-6372	www.surgeongeneral.gov/tobacco

Table 11 Internet Web-based Smoking Cessation Programs

Arizona Smokers' Help Line	http://www.ashline.org/quit/quitguide
Mayo Clinic	http://www.mayohealth.org/mayo/9910/htm/smoke.htm
Smoking Cessation Clinic at UCSF	http://www.stopsmoking.UCSF.edu/pages/index.asp

Figure 8 Fagerstrom Test for Nicotine Dependency

Question	Answers	Points
1. How soon after you wake up do you smoke your first cigarette?	Within 5 minutes Within 6 to 30 minutes	3 2
2. Do you find it difficult to refrain from smoking in places where it is forbidden, e.g., in church, at the library, in the cinema?	Yes No	1 0
3. Which cigarette would you hate most to give up?	The first in the morning All others	1 0
4. How many cigarettes per day do you smoke?	10 or fewer 11 to 20 21 to 30 31 or more	0 1 2 3
5. Do you smoke more frequently during the first hours after waking than during the rest of the day?	Yes No	1 0
6. Do you smoke even if you are so ill that you are in bed most of the day?	Yes No	1 0

Patients scoring 6 points or more are highly tobacco dependent and probably need nicotine replacement.

Physicians and the entire health team can motivate smokers to quit and teach them how to quit successfully. Many materials are available to help the primary care physician develop a program. The Agency for HealthCare Research and Quality (1-800-358-9295) publishes booklets and pamplets on the topic of smoking cessation for health professionals and the general public.

Other Causes of COPD

Certain industrial (e.g., isocyanates used in plastics and paints) and agricultural pollutants (e.g., grain dusts) have a small but causative role in the development of some COPD cases. These risk factors may be reduced by avoiding such substances when possible or wearing appropriate well-fitting masks, by increasing ventilation in work situations, and ultimately by calling for a reduction of these pollutants.

Conclusion

Prevention is the key to reducing and even eliminating COPD in the future. Public forums, including elementary schools, should be utilized by all physicians to spread the word that tobacco is a lethal substance. Many deadly diseases in addition to COPD, such as heart disease, vascular disease, and many cancers, result from tobacco smoking.

It has taken more than thirty years of aggressive action to spread the word about the dangers of tobacco use. The task is getting easier, and is finally meeting with some success in certain countries like the United States. Remind all patients that the substance that kills over 460,000 U.S. citizens each year is worthy of widespread discussion. Encourage them to participate actively in teaching young people never to start using tobacco. ■

References

Anda RF, Remington PL, Sienko DG, et al. Are physicians advising smokers to quit? The patient's perspective. JAMA 1987;257:1916-1919. This article gives evidence that patients do not perceive that their physicians are giving them strong advice to stop smoking.

Fiore MC, Baily WC, Cohen SJ, et al. A clinical practice guideline for treating tobacco use and dependence. A U.S. Public Health Service report. JAMA 2000; 283:3244-3253. A concensus statement of updated guidelines for brief and intensive tobacco cessation interventions. Assessment and treatment of tobacco use are also summarized.

Fiore MC, Smith SS, Jorenby DE, et al. The effectiveness of nicotine patch for smoking cessation. JAMA 1994;271:1940-1947. This classic meta-analysis strongly suggests the use of nicotine patches in virtually all smoking cessation clinics. Use of the patch greatly augments advice to quit smoking and other behavioral modification techniques.

Prochaska JO, DiClemente CC. Stages and processes of self-change of smoking: toward an integrative model of change. J Consult Clin Psychol 1983;51:390-395. Excellent smoking cessation guidelines.

Russell MAH, Wilson C, et al. Effect of general practitioners' advice against smoking. BMJ1979;2:231-235. A general description of a classic effective plan for smoking cessation.

U.S. Department of Health and Human Services. *Treating Tobacco Use and Dependence*. Public Health Service 2000. 179 pages. Clinical practice guidelines identify effective, experimentally validated tobacco dependence treatments and practices.

K. Consultation with a Pulmonary Specialist

One of the premises of this monograph is that the primary care physician should be able to diagnose and manage the great majority of patients with COPD throughout the course of their illness. There are several clinical circumstances, however, in which consultation with a pulmonary specialist is indicated. Patients with very severe disease accompanied by complications might best be managed in conjunction with a consultant.

Indications for Consultation

1. Particularly severe disease, including:
   a. persistent dyspnea with activities of daily living despite therapy, or
   b. frequent recurrent exacerbations.

Consultation on these patients may address:

- evaluation of other etiologies of dyspnea.
- review of the therapeutic regimen and recommendations for revisions or additional therapy.
- consideration of additional therapy for intractable dyspnea including possible use of codeine or narcotics (to partially blunt excessive respiratory drives).
- second opinion or discussion of advance directives, especially for subsequent severe exacerbations with acute respiratory failure, including discussion of withholding and/or withdrawing life support measures.

2. Evaluation for and initiation of maintenance oxygen therapy.
   - This includes consideration of nocturnal oxygen therapy for nocturnal hypoxemia and consideration of transtracheal oxygen therapy.

3. Failure to successfully taper the patient from systemic corticosteroids.

4. Consideration of and preoperative assessment for thoracic surgery and other surgery placing the patient at high risk for pulmonary complications.

5. Failure to respond after two courses of antibiotics for an acute exacerbation.

6. Presence of severe purulent chronic bronchitis or bronchiectasis for consideration of long-term intermittent or continuous antibiotic therapy.

7 Persistent pulmonary infiltrate(s) on chest radiograph unresponsive to a course of antibiotics.
   - This includes evaluation for tuberculosis, atypical mycobacterial disease, fungal disease, and lung cancer.

8. Evaluation of sleep disturbances, including suspected obstructive sleep apnea.

9. Management of severe acute respiratory failure.
   - This is particularly indicated if treatment with mechanical ventilation is a consideration.

10. Cor pulmonale with clinical right heart failure that is unresponsive to usual therapy.

11. Consideration of new techniques in lung volume reduction surgery.

12. Consideration for alpha-1- antitrypsin (Prolastin®) augmentation therapy. ■

L. Medicolegal Aspects

In the current climate of increasing medical litigation, it behooves every physician to be prudent in order to prevent legal action. The shift in responsibility for the management of more and more patients with COPD from pulmonary specialists to primary care physicians brings with it certain litigious pitfalls all should know. These are listed in Table 12. It should be emphasized that the corrective actions proposed are not self-serving, but actually improve the quality of patient care.

Perhaps the most frequent cause of medicolegal dispute –one that concerns all patients, not just those with COPD–is failure to adequately document all contact with and advice given to patients. Particular problems in this regard that do involve patients with COPD concern poor compliance with the treatment regimen, including failure to quit smoking, and side effects of drugs, especially long-term corticosteroids. Failure to hospitalize, failure to refer for consultation, and failure to recognize non-COPD pulmonary diseases or COPD-associated complications are other potential causes of litigation that are dealt with elsewhere in this monograph. ■

Table 12 Potential Medicolegal Issues

Important problems in the management of COPD that may lead to medicolegal action.

Potential Problem	Solution
Use of drugs, especially long-term corticosteroids.	Discuss with patient and document. Provide list of possible side effects. Obtain consent for dangerous drugs. Consult to affirm need.
Noncompliance with regimen, including failure to quit smoking	Discuss with patient and document. Send letter.
Failure to hospitalize.	See Section H.4. Consult to clarify.
Failure to refer.	See Section K.
Failure to recognize other disorders (tuberculosis and cancer) or complications (cor pulmonale and respiratory failure).	Be aware of possibilities indentified in Sections H.1-H.5 Consult to clarify.

M. The National Lung Health Education Program, (NLHEP)

A new national healthcare initiative known as the National Lung Health Education Program, (NLHEP), is directed at COPD and related disorders, including lung cancer, heart attack, and stroke. Thus, this is a new initiative for improved general health in America. The key role of the primary care physician and respiratory care practitioners is stressed by the NLHEP. The NLHEP is directed to all primary care practitioners, the public, third party payers, and healthcare administrators. The NLHEP urges that all primary care physicians and other healthcare providers obtain simple, accurate, handheld spirometers for office and clinic use. Only the FEV_1 and the FVC are required to assess patients with COPD in incipient or advanced stages of disease. "Test Your Lungs, Know Your Numbers" is the battle cry of the NLHEP. ■

N. Postscript and Biographical Sketches of Authors

Frontline Treatment of COPD is intended to be a primer for primary care physicians. The authors believe that they have provided a timely and succinct message that can help primary care physicians immediately improve treatment for patients with COPD. Unfortunately, every detail of the management of COPD could not be included in a book of this size and scope. Also, new conceptual and technological advances, including new pharmacological agents and drug-delivery devices, are anticipated in the future.

Finally, let us offer an innovative philosophy–based entirely on clinical studies–about the basic nature of COPD. Whether or not this hypothesis explains the multiplicity of factors that conspire to create the pathophysiological state of COPD–a process which takes 30 to 40 years and culminates with premature morbidity and mortality–remains to be established.

It may be appropriate to consider COPD as a multi-system disease. Patients with any stage of COPD exhibit a common affective disorder that is characterized by anxiety, depression, and somatic preoccupation. Anxiety and depression can be reduced with tobacco use, which may be one of the main reasons why nicotine addiction in COPD patients is so strong. In addition, smokers weigh less than nonsmokers. They tend to consume foods higher in fat and cholesterol and lower in fiber and antioxidant vitamins. Deficiency in antioxidant vitamins may be an additional factor in the premature morbidity and mortality suffered by COPD patients. Accordingly, the treatment of COPD may take on a new conceptual framework when we consider that COPD may, in fact, be a systemic illness. ■

(continued)

References

Petty TL (editorial). Pulmonary rehabilitation of early COPD: COPD as a systemic disease. Chest 1994;105:1636-1637. COPD should be considered a systemic disease and pulmonary rehabilitation should be provided for patients in all stages of disease.

Editor

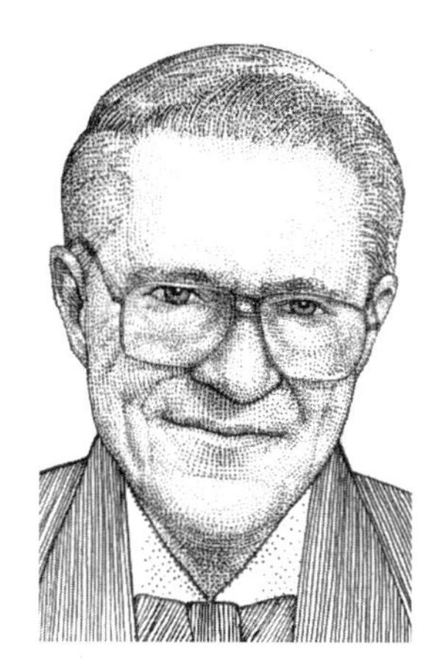

Thomas L. Petty, M.D.

Thomas L. Petty, M.D. received his M.D. at the University of Colorado in 1958. He interned at Philadelphia General Hospital and received his residency training at the University of Michigan and the University of Colorado. His pulmonary training was at the University of Colorado. He is a pulmonologist and Professor of Medicine at the University of Colorado Health Sciences Center in Denver and at Rush University in Chicago. He was previously head of the Division of Pulmonary Sciences at the University and Director of the Fellowship Training Program.

Dr. Petty was founding President of the Association of Pulmonary Program Directors, (APPD), and has served as President of the American College of Chest Physicians. He is a former member of the Board of Governors of the American Board of Internal Medicine.

Dr. Petty has received the Distinguished Service Award of the American Thoracic Society (1995), elected to the Colorado Pulmonary Physicians' "Hall of Fame" (1995) and received the annual award for excellence by the American Association for Respiratory and Cardiovascular Rehabilitation (1995). He was elected to Master Fellow of the American College of Chest Physicians (1995). He also received the Master Award of the American College of Physicians in 1996.
Dr. Petty has been named Chairman of the National Lung Health Education Program, (NLHEP). Its goal is the early diagnosis of COPD and lung cancer.

Today, Dr. Petty also remains active in teaching, patient care, and research. He enjoys fishing, small game hunting, and playing with his three "kids" and eight grandchildren.

(continued)

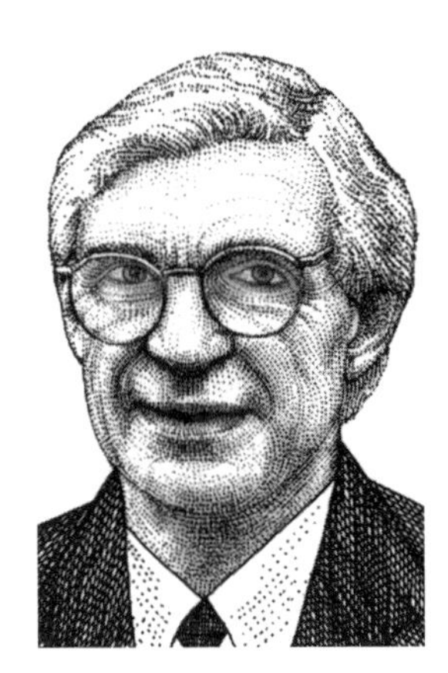

J. Roy Duke, Jr., M.D.
Dr. Duke was born in Ocala, Florida and attended Tulane University School of Medicine in New Orleans, Louisiana, obtaining his medical degree in 1960. After a two-year stint in the U.S. Air Force, he completed his postgraduate training in pulmonary medicine at Tulane in 1967.

Dr. Duke joined the Palm Beach Medical Group in West Palm Beach, Florida in 1967 and has practiced pulmonary medicine and internal medicine there to the present. He has served as Chief of Medicine and Chief of Staff of Good Samaritan Hospital in West Palm Beach and is currently the Director of Pulmonary Services.

He has an interest in Hyperbaric Medicine, which is an extension of his hobbies of scuba diving and underwater photography. He is also an avid fly fisherman and fly tier. Dr. Duke is married to Bobbye Craig Duke and has two children, Denise and Christopher.

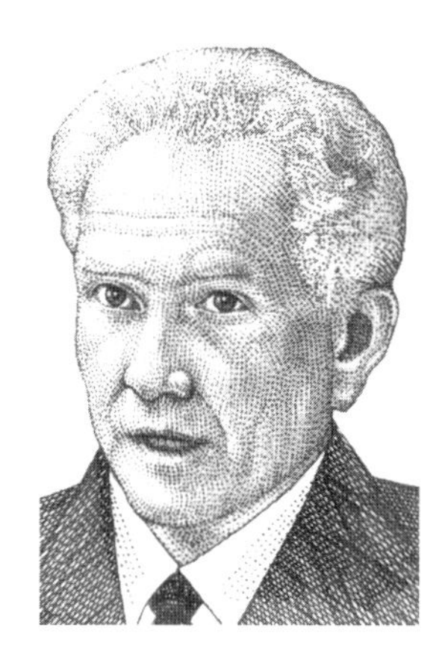

James T. Good, Jr., M.D.

Dr. Good received his M.D. degree from the University of Kansas and then completed a medical internship, residency and chief medical residency also at the University of Kansas. He then completed a three-year pulmonary and critical care fellowship at the University of Colorado. The next four years he remained on the faculty at the University of Colorado as an Assistant Professor of Medicine and was Medical Director of both the Respiratory Therapy Department and the Critical Care Unit at Denver General Hospital.

His scientific interests include management of critical patients with acute respiratory failure, pleural diseases and asthma. He is a fellow of the American College of Physicians and the American College of Chest Physicians, and served as the Governor for the states of Colorado and Wyoming for the ACCP from 1988 to 1994.

He currently is in the private practice of pulmonary and critical care medicine in south Denver and is Medical Director of the Swedish/Columbia Critical Care Unit. He remains actively involved in clinical research, teaching medical students and residents, and in continuing medical education programs.

(continued)

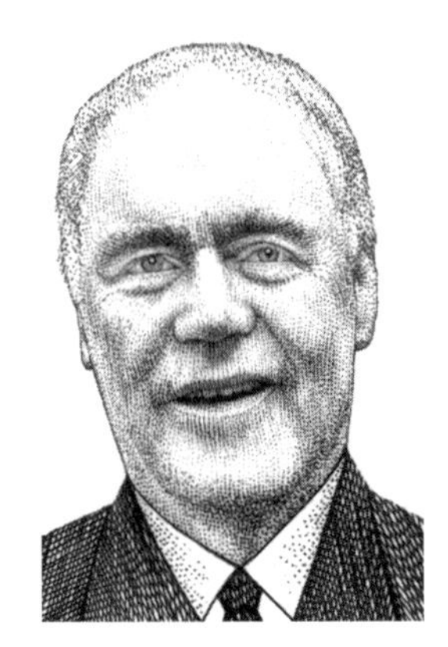

Leonard D. Hudson, M.D.

Dr. Hudson received his B.S. from Washington State University in Pullman, Washington and his M.D. from the University of Washington, Seattle. He did his internship at Bellevue Hospital Center (New York) and his residency at New York Hospital, Cornell Medical Center (New York) and at the University of Washington (Seattle). From 1971 to 1973, Dr. Hudson was an attending physician at Colorado General Hospital in Denver. In 1973, he moved to the Harborview Medical Center in Seattle, where he rose to Associate Physician-in-Chief in the Department of Medicine.

In 1985, Dr. Hudson became Head of Pulmonary and Critical Care Medicine at the University of Washington. Since 1982, he has been a Professor of Medicine at the University of Washington, Seattle.

Dr. Hudson's honors include Outstanding Resident, Harborview Medical Center; American Thoracic Society Fellowship in Pulmonary Diseases; Chair, Pulmonary Disease Subspecialty Board, American Board of Internal Medicine; and Chair, Critical Care Medicine Test Committee, American Board of Internal Medicine.
He was President of the American Thoracic Society from 1995 to 1996.

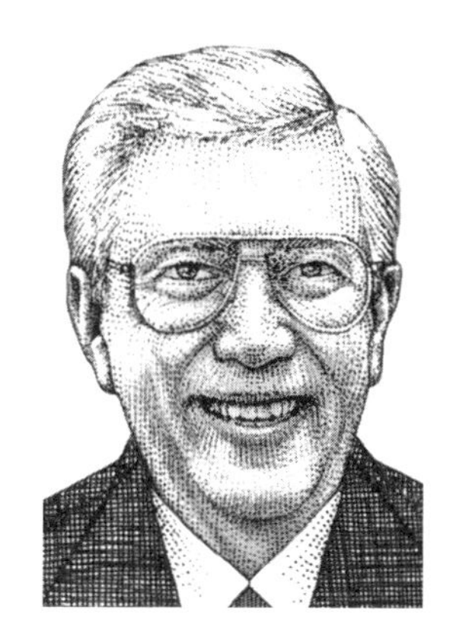

Dean D. Mergenthaler, M.D.

Dr. Mergenthaler has an undergraduate degree in chemistry and biology from Cornell University, a Master's degree in human anatomy from the University of Miami School of Medicine, a medical doctor degree from Jefferson Medical College, with internship at Robert Packer Guthrie Hospital and Clinic and internal medicine residency and pulmonary fellowship at Jackson Memorial Hospital.

Dr. Mergenthaler has been in private practice of pulmonary and internal medicine for the past 30 years in Palm Beach County, Florida. He has been active in the development and medical directorship of several hospital Respiratory Therapy Departments, as well as in the development of a local community medical center.

His hobbies include fishing, traveling, reading, and gardening. He and his wife, Mary Beth, have two grown children.

(continued)

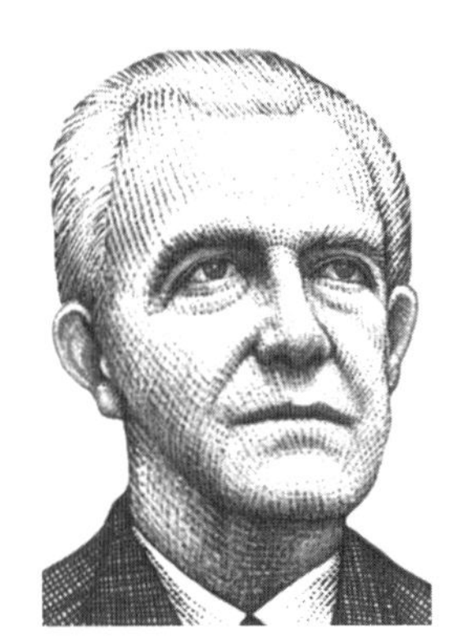

John F. Murray, M.D.

After receiving his B.A. (1949) and M.D. (1953) degrees, both from Stanford University, Dr. Murray had two years of medical residency training at San Francisco General Hospital and two more years at Kings County Hospital (New York). Afterward, he had a year of research training at the Royal Postgraduate Medical School in London.

He started his faculty career at the University of California, Los Angeles in 1957, rising to the rank of Associate Professor of Medicine and Physiology. In 1966 he moved to the University of California, San Francisco, where he became Professor of Medicine in 1969. He was also a member of the Senior Staff of the Cardiovascular Research Institute and Chief of the Chest Service at San Francisco General Hospital (1966 to 1989).

He became Professor Emeritus in 1994, and now works mainly in Paris, France as President (1992 to 1996) of the International Union Against Tuberculosis and Lung Disease. Dr. Murray received the College Medal of the American College of Chest Physicians (1985), the Trudeau Medal of the American Thoracic Society (1989), and the President's Award of the European Respiratory Society (1996).

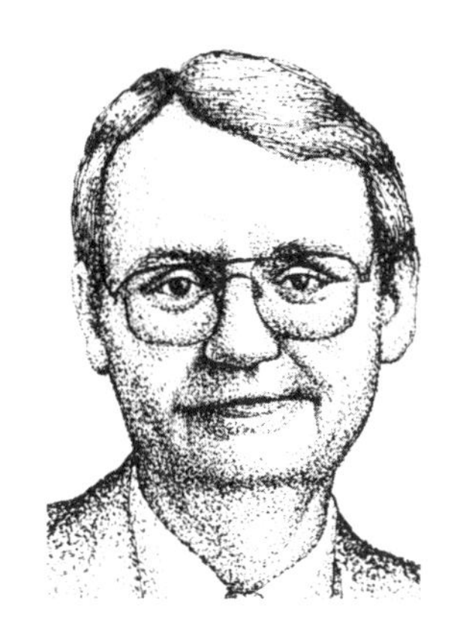

Thomas A. Neff, M.D. (1937–1994)
Dr. Neff was a Professor of Medicine and served as Chief of Denver General Hospital's Pulmonary and Critical Care Medicine Service as well as Denver General Hospital's Medical Director of Respiratory Care for 25 years. He graduated from Northwestern University School of Medicine in 1963 and served a year at the Army's 85th Evacuation Hospital in Vietnam. He joined the Colorado Pulmonary fellowship training program in 1967. After finishing his training, he joined the University of Colorado Health Sciences Center and eventually became head of Pulmonary Services at Denver General Hospital. He worked diligently to build an excellent educational environment for many of today's national leaders in pulmonary diseases. He participated in many clinical trials and took a leadership role in the Oxygen Consensus Conferences organized by the Denver group. Dr. Neff was dedicated to excellence in patient care. Truly one of the leaders in pulmonary medicine, Dr. Neff died in December, 1994 of cancer.

(continued)

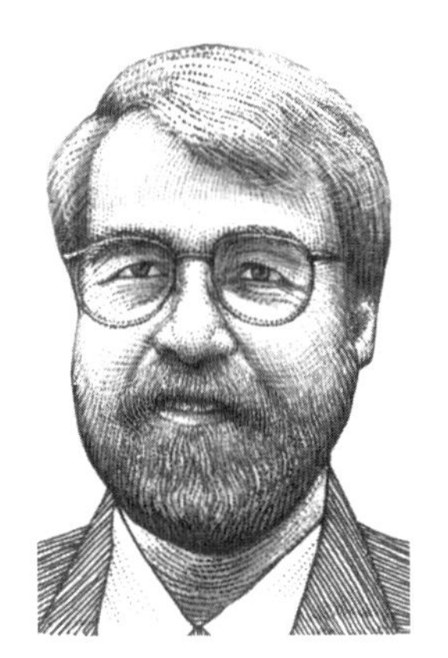

Donald R. Rollins, M.D.

Dr. Rollins is a pulmonologist who was engaged in clinical practice in Loveland, Colorado, for 22 years, where he was Medical Director of the Cardiopulmonary Department at McKee Medical Center. He is a Fellow of the American College of Chest Physicians and he is an Associate Clinical Professor in the Pulmonary Division at the University of Colorado Health Sciences Center in Denver and continues to be actively involved with clinical research. Dr. Rollins received his B.A. at St. Olaf College and his M.D. from the University of North Carolina. He did his internship, residency and pulmonary fellowship at the University of Texas. Dr. Rollins has recently joined the Greenbrier Clinic in White Sulphur Springs, West Virginia.

He enjoys fishing with friends and playing string bass and guitar with his daughter Elizabeth and wife Susan, both accomplished musicians. ■

O. The Snowdrift Pulmonary Conference

A small group of pulmonologists and their colleagues from industry comprise the Snowdrift Pulmonary Conference. We meet once a year to exchange our experiences and philosophies about the care of our patients, who suffer from a variety of pulmonary disorders.

During the Conference, we voice our beliefs and our disagreements with equal fervor. Always, we indulge in a spiritual feeling of great friendship.

We hope that our words of advice and occasional wisdom will be appreciated by all who read them. We offer them to you in a spirit of fellowship and love for our patients. ■

On Wisdom:

> *A sadder and wiser man*
> *He rose the morrow morn*
>
> S.T. Coleridge, The Ancient Mariner

On Snowdrift:

> *If winter comes, can*
> *Spring be far behind*
>
> Shelley, Ode to the West Wind

Appendix A Comprehensive Respiratory Screening Form

IDENTIFICATION DATA Fill in the following information as it relates to you. PLEASE PRINT.

Name ______________________ Date __________ # __________

Address ______________________ Date of Birth __________

______________________ (zip code) ___Married ___Separated ___Divorced ___Widowed ___Single

Home Telephone ______________________ (area code)

Education: ___years Elementary ___years High School ___years College, Technical, Business, etc.

Employer ______________________

Business Telephone ______________________ (area code)

Occupation ______________________

SPECIAL PROBLEMS OR SYMPTOMS

1. In the blank lines below, please describe any special problems or symptoms you would like to discuss with the doctor today:

____

____

____

____

2. How long have you had this problem? . . . . ___for 1 week ___for 1 month ___for 1 year ___over 1 year
3. Have you ever seen a doctor for this problem in the past? . . . . ___Yes ___No

IF YES: a. How did the doctor diagnose your problem? ______________________

____

b. How did the doctor treat your problem? ______________________

____

c Did the treatment help you? . . . . ___Yes ___No

GENERAL SCREEN

1. Please place an (X) next to any of the following problems that you have right now:

___frequent headaches
___trouble with eyes or vision
___trouble with ears or hearing
___trouble with nose
___congested nose or nose bleeds
___trouble smelling
___coughing spells
___coughing up a lot of phlegm
___trouble breathing (shortness of breath)
___dizzy spells

___trouble with stomach or digestion
___vomiting
___trouble with bowels
___constipation
___loose bowels
___blood in stools
___trouble with urination
___difficulty starting urine
___trouble with genitals
___trouble with periods

___trouble with bruises
___aching muscles or joints
___numbness in fingers
___crying spells
___work or family problems
___sexual difficulties
___fever
___weight changes
___fatigue

2. Have you ever considered committing suicide? ____Yes ____No
3. Have you ever used marijuana or heroin, LSD, or similar drugs? ____Yes ____No
4. Are you allergic to any medications, foods or other substances? ____Yes ____No
   IF YES, what? ____
5. List all medications you are currently taking: ____
6. When is the last time you had a physical examination? ____Year
7. Have you ever been told you had any chronic or serious illness? ____Yes ____No
   IF YES, please list the illnesses you have now or have had: ____

8. Give the following information for the last three times you have been hospitalized starting with the most recent. (Do not list normal pregnancies.)

	HOSPITALIZATION (1)	HOSPITALIZATION (2)	HOSPITALIZATION (3)
Type of operation or illness:			
Month and year hospitalized:			
Name of hospital:			
City and State:			

9. Please list the following information for your blood relatives:

	Year of Birth	Major Illnesses		If dead, age at death and cause. Age	Cause
Father					
Mother					
Brothers or Sisters					

CONTINUE TO NEXT PAGE

(Do not write below this line. For doctor's notes.)

continued

Please answer each of the following questions by placing an (X) in the blank at the right that most applies to you. If you are unable to answer a question for any reason, place a solid circle (●) in the first blank.

1. .... Has anyone in your family had lung disease?	**1. __Yes __No**
2. ...... Has anyone in your family ever had asthma, hayfever or chronic bronchitis?	**2. __Yes __No**
3. .... Has anyone in your family had allergies?	**3. __Yes __No**
4. .... Are you allergic to any drugs?	**4. __Yes __No**
IF YES: .... Please list the drugs you are allergic to in the blank space at the right:	__________ __________
5. .... Were you ever allergic to milk?	**5. __Yes __No**
6. .... Are you now allergic to any foods?	**6. __Yes __No**
IF YES: ...... Please list the foods you are allergic to in the blank spaces to the right:	__________ __________
7. .... Have you ever been treated for asthma?	**7. __Yes __No**
8. .... Have you ever been treated for hayfever?	**8. __Yes __No**
9. .... Have you ever been treated for intestinal parasites?	**9. __Yes __No**
10. .... Do you have any other allergies?	**10. __Yes __No**
IF YES: .... Please list them in the blank spaces at the right:	__________ __________
11. **Have you ever had any of the following illnesses:**	**11.**
a. .... a chest operation	**a. __Yes __No**
b. .... a chest injury	**b. __Yes __No**
c. .... broken ribs	**c. __Yes __No**
d. .... sinus trouble	**d. __Yes __No**
e. .... pneumonia	**e. __Yes __No**
f. .... pleurisy	**f. __Yes __No**
g. .... emphysema	**g. __Yes __No**
h. .... fungus disease of the lung	**h. __Yes __No**
i. .... lung cancer	**i. __Yes __No**
j. .... collapsed lung	**j. __Yes __No**
12. .... Have you ever had tuberculosis (T.B.)?	**12. __Yes __No**
13. .... Have you been exposed to someone with active tuberculosis?	**13. __Yes __No**
14. .... Have you ever had a positive T.B. skin test?	**14. __Yes __No**
15. .... Have you had a chest x-ray in the past year?	**15. __Yes __No**
16. .... Have you ever had an abnormal chest x-ray?	**16. __Yes __No**
17. .... Have you ever had a breathing (blowing) test?	**17. __Yes __No**
18. .... Have you ever had an abnormal breathing test?	**18. __Yes __No**

19. .... Have you ever had air put into your chest or abdomen as a treatment?	19. ___Yes ___No
20. Have you ever lived in any of the following places:	20.
a. .... Arizona	a. ___Yes ___No
b. .... Ohio Valley	b. ___Yes ___No
c. .... the South	c. ___Yes ___No
21. .... Have you ever traveled through or lived in Southern California?	21. ___Yes ___No
IF YES: .... Did you get sick with a sudden flu-like illness while there?	___Yes ___No
22. .... Have you been abroad in the last 5 years?	22. ___Yes ___No
IF YES: .... List the countries you visited in the blank spaces at the right:	____________________
	____________________
23. .... Have you ever been a metal worker?	23. ___Yes ___No
24. .... Have you ever worked in a foundry?	24. ___Yes ___No
25. .... Have you ever been a welder?	25. ___Yes ___No
26. .... Have you ever worked in any mines?	26. ___Yes ___No
27. .... Have you ever been a stone quarry worker?	27. ___Yes ___No
28. .... Have you ever worked as a farmer?	28. ___Yes ___No
29. .... Have you ever worked as a plumber?	29. ___Yes ___No
30. .... Have you ever worked with or been exposed to asbestos?	30. ___Yes ___No
31. .... Have you ever been exposed to moldy wheat or wheat dust?	31. ___Yes ___No
32. .... Have you ever worked with or been exposed to beryllium?	32. ___Yes ___No
33. .... Have you ever been in contact with anyone who had beryllium poisoning?	33. ___Yes ___No
34. .... Do you have any pets?	34. ___Yes ___No
IF YES: a. .... Do you have any cats?	a. ___Yes ___No
b. .... Do you have any dogs?	b. ___Yes ___No
c. .... Do you have any birds?	c. ___Yes ___No
d. .... Do you own any pigeons?	d. ___Yes ___No

continued

35. Do you have a cough?	35. ___Yes ___No
IF YES: a. How long have you had a cough?	a. ___for 1 month ___for 1 year ___over 1 year
b. How often do you have a cough?	b. ___almost always ___often ___sometimes
c. How severe has your cough been?	c. ___severe ___moderately severe ___mild
d. When do you cough most often?	d. ___when lying down ___when arising in the morning ___at night ___during the day
e. Do you bring up phlegm or mucus each day?	e. ___Yes ___No
IF YES: (1) What color is the phlegm you bring up?	(1) ___greenish ___white and foamy ___gray and foamy ___bloody
(2) Do you have to cough more than 5 times to clear your throat of phlegm?	(2) ___Yes ___No
(3) Do you bring up phlegm when arising from bed?	(3) ___Yes ___No
36. During the past 3 years have you coughed up phlegm for 3 or more weeks at a time?	36. ___Yes ___No
37. Have you ever coughed up blood?	37. ___Yes ___No
38. Do you have a cold now?	38. ___Yes ___No
39. How many colds a year do you get?	39. ___colds per year
40. Do you get more colds during the winter than in the summer?	40. ___Yes ___No
41. Do your colds always seem to settle in your chest?	41. ___Yes ___No
42. Do you have difficulty shaking off a cold?	42. ___Yes ___No
43. Are you troubled with hoarseness?	43. ___Yes ___No
IF YES: a. How long has this been happening?	a. ___for 1 month ___for 1 year ___over 1 year
b. Have you had hoarseness that began after a thyroid (goiter) operation?	b. ___Yes ___No
44. Do you have shortness of breath?	44. ___Yes ___No
IF YES: a. How long has this been happening?	a. ___for 1 month ___for 1 year ___over 1 year
b. How often has this been happening?	b. ___daily ___weekly ___monthly
c. How severe has your shortness of breath been?	c. ___severe ___moderately severe ___mild
d. When do you get short of breath?	d. ___when climbing stairs ___when just walking on level ground ___walking up a slight hill ___walking with people your own age ___sleeping in bed

45. .... Do you have wheezing or whistling sounds when you breathe? 45. ___Yes ___No
IF YES: a. .... How long has this been happening? a. ___for 1 month ___for 1 year ___over 1 year
b. .... How often has this been happening? b. ___daily ___weekly ___monthly
c. .... How severe has your wheezing been? c. ___severe ___moderately severe ___mild
d. .... Do you wheeze when you exert yourself? d. ___Yes ___No
e. .... Do you cough when you exert yourself? e. ___Yes ___No

46. **Have you ever had stabbing chest pains that worsened when you took a deep breath?** 46. ___Yes ___No

47. .... Do you awaken at night in a sweat? 47. ___Yes ___No
IF YES: a. .... How long has this been happening? a. ___for 1 month ___for 1 year ___over 1 year
b. .... How often has this been happening? b. ___daily ___weekly ___monthly
c. .... How severe has this sweating been? c. ___severe ___moderately severe ___mild

48. .... Do you have a tendency to sneeze in the morning? 48. ___Yes ___No

49. .... Have you had a problem with diarrhea or frothy stools? 49. ___Yes ___No

50. **Do you smoke any of the following:** 50.
a. .... cigarettes? a. ___Yes ___No
b. .... a pipe? b. ___Yes ___No
c. .... cigars? c. ___Yes ___No

51. If you smoke cigarettes, how much do you smoke: 51.
a. .... less than 10 a day? a. ___Yes ___No
b. .... between 10 and 20 a day? b. ___Yes ___No
c. .... between 20 and 40 a day? c. ___Yes ___No
d. .... over 2 packs a day? d. ___Yes ___No

52. If you smoke cigarettes, how long have you been smoking at your present rate: 52. ___Yes ___No
a. .... for about a month? a. ___Yes ___No
b. .... for about a year? b. ___Yes ___No
c. .... for several years? c. ___Yes ___No

53. .... If you do not smoke now, did you ever smoke? 53. ___Yes ___No
IF YES, write in the year when you stopped: ___________year stopped

end of form

A

B

C

F

G

H

I

L

O

P

T

V